INTRODUCTION

Medical terminology is becoming more and more main stream, as health care becomes the responsibility of the patient. So what does that term mean, QUICKLY!!

This whole area can be very confusing as approximately 75% of medical terminology is either Greek - for diseases & disease processes, or Latin -major organs & their related systems. However this protocol is not always followed and many other terms is eponymous, named after the discoverer, or eminent scientist in the field, and increasingly more abbreviated. Medical terms are difficult to understand, spell and pronounce, and may mean one thing in one specialty but another in a different health / medical area. This book is a guide through this maze. It is not only a dictionary but rather a guide through common medical terms and a HOW TO book. **How to construct and de-construct the meaning of medial terms.** They cannot all be listed and new ones are constantly appearing: new diseases are discovered; new processes mapped out. Tables of the word prefixes, suffixes, and word roots are placed at the beginning of the book, to help in this process.

Lists and Tables of ba ... and
means of specimen p ... placed
after a person's name ... and
other academic forur ... ical,
science, etiquette bo

The A to Zs are incr ... ew
book there is a new
pathological as the series enters a new phase of the *A to Z of the Failure of...* series – the first of which is the *A to Z of Bone and Joint Failure.*

If there is a structure / subject you want to see in the A to Zs let us know. anatomy.update@gmail.com

We have 2 websites and there maybe others where you can view all images of the A to Zs and any additional material please feel free to examine the new books which may be placed here and to give any suggestions. The order of the new titles is often guided by the feedback received. http://www.aspenpharma.com.au/atlas/student.htm www.amandasatoz.com

ACKNOWLEDGEMENT

hank you Aspenpharmacare Australia for your support and assistance in this valuable project, particularly Mr. Greg Lan, and Rob Koster. Thank you to all those who have helped when I have been rushed to finish and have made time for this project, and have faith in it, in particular Ante Mihaljevic and Phill Ryman. Thank you everyone who has provided valuable feedback, and help in many ways; Richard, Peter, Robbie, Jody, Quentin and my own A to Z the alphabet of my life - there are others too, thank you.

DEDICATION

To people who love words – onomatophilics, and want to use them well. Let's have words, words and more words!!!

HOW TO USE THIS BOOK

The Table of Contents as usual guides the reader through this book's sections – within which the subject is listed alphabetically.
The elements of a typical medical term – COMPOUND WORD - are –

The Prefix	Combining Vowel	Word Root	Combining Vowel	The Suffix

The main text lists the word roots prefixes and suffixes with the Greek or Latin etc meaning, the common explanation of the **ANATOMICAL term is in RED** unless it is a PATHOLOGICAL term where it is in GREEN.
Pronunciation guides are alongside terms where necessary, as well as a listing of the common forms of the word roots: adjectives plurals etc.
Note there may be more than one of each element present but they are not necessarily always present in each term.
As well as this a guide lists all these word components in a table form before the main text. Word roots with their prefix and suffix forms are in BLUE in both sections. Combining vowels of "A" "O" etc used to make pronunciation easier are not listed with the term but added in the compound word.
PREFIXES are generally used to further describe the term indicating: amount, colour, direction, location, number & negation i.e. the absence of, position, or time.
SUFFIXES are generally used to modify the basic word indicating: condition, disease, procedure, or part of speech e.g. adjective etc
ABBREVIATIONS are used increasingly often replacing the original term, in common use. These have been placed in a separate section. Some are also placed alongside the term itself in the main text.

Thank you

A. L. Neill
BSc MSc MBBS PhD FACBS
medicalamanda@gmail.com
ISBN 978-1-921930-01-0

Table of contents

Anatomical, Medical and Clinical Abbreviations and Acronyms in common use

A

A = actions movements of a joint
a = artery
aa = anastomoses
AA = amino acids / androgenic alopecia
AAA = abdominal aortic aneurysm
AAD = antibiotic-associated diarrhoea
AAO = alert, awake, and orientated
A&O = alert & orientated
Ab = antibody = IL
Ab/Ag = antigen antibody complex
ABD/Abd = abdomen
ABG = arterial blood gas
AC = before eating
ACD = acute contact dermatitis
ACLS = advanced cardiac life support
ACTH = adrenocorticotropic hormone
ad libitum/ad lib = take as needed / no restrictions
ADD = attention deficit disorder
ADH = anti-diuretic hormone
ADHD = attention deficit hyperactivity disorder
adj. = adjective
ADR = adverse drug reaction / acute dystonic reaction
AED = antiepileptic drug
AF = atrial fibrillation / afebrile
AFB = acid-fast bacilli
AFP = alpha-fetoprotein
AFX = atypical fibroxanthoma
A /G = albumin/globulin ratio
Ag = antigen
AI = aortic insufficiency
AI = acute inflammation
AK = actinic keratosis
AKA = above the knee amputation
aka = also known as
ALD = alcoholic liver disease
ALL = acute lymphocytic leukaemia
alt. = alternative
Amb = ambulate
AML = acute myelogenous leukaemia
ANA = antinuclear antibody
ANF = antinuclear factor
ANS = autonomic nervous system
ant. = anterior
AOB = alcohol on breath
AODM = adult onset diabetes mellitus
AP = anteroposterior or abdominal - perineal
AR = allergic reaction
ARDS = acute respiratory distress syndrome
ARF = acute renal failure
art. = articulation, artery
AS = aortic stenosis
AS = Alternative spelling, generally referring to the differences b/n British and American spelling
ASAP = as soon as possible
ASCVD = atherosclerotic cardiovascular disease
ASD = atrial septal defect
ASHD = atherosclerotic heart disease
AST = anal skin tag
AV = atrioventricular
A-V = arteriovenous
A-VO2 = arteriovenous oxygen

B

b/n = between
BBB bundle branch block / blood brain barrier
bc = because
BCAA = branched chain amino acids
BCC = basal cell carcinoma
BCR = B-cell antigen receptor
bd/bid = twice a day
BD = Bowen's disease / twice daily
BE = barium enema
BEE = basal energy expenditure
BF = blood flow
BKA = below the knee amputation
BLK = benign lichenoid keratosis / benign lymphocytic keratosis
BL = basal lamina
BM = bone marrow /bowel movement/basement membrane
bm = basement membrane
BMR = basal metabolic rate
b/n = between
BOM = bilateral otitis media
BP = blood pressure / bullous pemphigoid
BPH = benign prostatic hypertrophy
BPM = beats per minute
BRBPR = bright red blood per rectum
BRP = bathroom privileges
BS = bowel sounds / breath sounds / blood stream / blood supply
BUN = blood urea nitrogen
BV(s) = blood vessel(s)
BV = blood vessels
BW = body weight
Bx = biopsy

C

c = with
C = carpal / cervical
CA = cancer/carcinoma
Ca = calcium /carcinoma
CAA = crystalline amino acids
CABG = coronary artery bypass graft
CAD = coronary artery disease
CAT (scan) = computerized axial tomography
CBC = complete blood count
CBG = capillary blood gas
CC = cervical cortex
CC = chief complaint
CCF = chronic cardiac failure
CCU = cardiac care unit
CCV = critical closing volume
CD = cluster of differentiation
c.f. = as demonstrated / that means
CF = cystic fibrosis
CFU = colony forming unit
C&S = culture and sensitivity
CGL = chronic granulocytic leukaemia
CHF = congestive heart failure
CHO = carbohydrate
chol. = cholesterol
CI = cardiac index
CIf = chronic inflammation
CIN = carcinoma in situ
CK = creatinine kinase
cm = cell membrane
CML = chronic myelogenous leukaemia
CMV = cytomegalovirus
CN = cranial nerves / compound naevus
CNS = central nervous system
CO = cardiac output
C/O = complaining of
Co = coccygeal / collagen
COAD = chronic obstructive airways disease
coag. = coagulation
COLD = chronic obstructive lung disease
COPD = chronic obstructive pulmonary disease

C *continued*

CONN = congenital naevus
CP = cerebral palsy / cervical plexus / chest pain
CP = chest pain/cerebral palsy
CPAP = continuous positive airway pressure
CPDN = compound naevus
CPK = creatinine phosphokinase
CPR = cardiopulmonary resuscitation
Cr = cranial
CRCL = creatinine clearance
CRF = chronic renal failure
CRP = C-reactive protein
CSF = Cerebrospinal fluid / colony stimulating factor
CSSD = chronic superficial scaling dermatitis
CT = connective tissue / computerized tomography
CTCL = cutaneous T cell lymphoma
cut. = cutaneous
CUT HORN = cutaneous horn
CVA = cerebrovascular accident /costovertebral angle
CVAT = tenderness at the costovertebral angle
CVP = central venous pressure
CX = cicatrix
CXR/CX = chest X-ray

D

DA = dermatitis artifacta
DAT = diet as tolerated
DAW = dispense as written
DC = discontinue /discharge
D&C = dilation and curettage
DDx = differential diagnosis
DF = dermatofibroma
DFSP = dermatofibrosarcoma protuberans
D5W = 5% dextrose in water
DH = dermatitis herpetiformis
DHT = dihydrotestosterone
DI = diabetes insipidus
DIC = disseminated intravascular coagulopathy
DIF = direct immunofluorescence
diff. = difference(s)
DIP = distal interphalangeal joint
DJD = degenerative joint disease
DKA = diabetic ketoacidosis
dL/dl = decilitre
DLE = discoid lupus erythematosis
DM = diabetes mellitus
DMS = dermatomyositis
DN = dermal naevus
DNR = do not resuscitate
DNS = did not survive processing (e.g. tissue sample)
DOA = dead on arrival
DOE = dyspnea on exertion
DPL = diagnostic peritoneal lavage
DPT = diphtheria, pertussis, tetanus
DRE = digital rectal examination
Ds = disease
DSAP = disseminated superficial actinic porokeratosis
DTR = deep tendon reflexes
DVT = deep venous thrombosis
DX = diagnosis
Dysp = dysplastic

E

EAA = essential amino acids
EAC = erythema annular centrificum
EAM = external acoustic meatus
EAS = external anal sphincter
EBA = epidermolysis bullosa acquisita
EBL = estimated blood loss
EC = extracellular (outside the cell)
ECG = electrocardiogram
ECT = electroconvulsive therapy
EED = erythema elevatum diutinum
EEG = electroencephalogram
EFAD = essential fatty acid deficiency
e.g. = example
EM = electron microscopy
EMG = electromyogram
EMS = erythema multiforma
EMV = eyes, motor, verbal response (Glasgow coma scale)
ENT = ears, nose, and throat
EOM = extraocular muscles
ESR = erythrocyte sedimentation rate
ER = extensor retinaculum
ET = endotracheal
ETT = endotracheal tube
ERCP = endoscopic retrograde cholangio-pancreatography
ETOH = ethanol
EUA = examination under anaesthesia
Ex = examination
ext. = extensor (as in muscle to extend across a joint)

F

Fab = antibody binding fragment
FB = foreign body
FBS = fasting blood sugar
Fc = fragment -crystallizable region
FDE = fixed drug eruption
FEV = forced expiratory volume
FFP = fresh frozen plasma
FFFT = fits, faints and/or funny turns
FR = flexor retinaculum
FRC = functional residual capacity
FTT = failure to thrive
FU = follow-up
FUO = fever of unknown origin
FVC = forced vital capacity
Fx = fracture

G

GA = granuloma annulare
GC = Gonorrhoea
GD = Grover's disease
GETT = general by endotracheal tube
GF = growth factors
GFR = glomerular filtration rate
GH = growth hormone
GI = gastrointestinal
GIT = gastrointestinal tract
Gk. = Greek
gld = gland
g/gm = gram
gr = grain; 1 grain = 65mg. Therefore Vgr = 325mg
grp = group
GSW = gun shot wound
Gt/gtt = drops
GTT = glucose tolerance test
GU = genitourinary
GVDH = graft versus host disease
GXT = graded exercise tolerance test (Stress test)

H

H = hormone
HA = headache
HAA = hepatitis B surface antigen
HAV = hepatitis A virus
Hb = haemoglobin
HBP = high blood pressure
HCG = human chorionic gonadotropin
HCT = hematocrit
HDL = high density lipoprotein
HEENT = head, eyes, ears, nose and throat
Hg = haemorrage
Hgb = haemoglobin
H/H = haemoglobin/haematocrit
HIV = human immunodeficiency virus
HK = solar keratosis
HLA = histocompatibility locus antigen
HMF = Hutchinson's melanotic freckle
HJR = hepatojugular reflex
HO = history of
HOB = head of bed
HP = high power
HPF = high power field
HPV = human papilloma virus
HPI = history of present illness
HR = heart rate
HS = at bedtime
HSM = hepatosplenomegaly
HSP = herpes simplex virus
HTLV-III = human lymphotropic virus, type III AIDS agent, HIV)
HSV = herpes simplex virus
HTN = hypertension
Hx = history

I

I = insertion
IAM = internal acoustic meatus
IAS = internal anal sphincter
I&D = incision and drainage
I&O = intake and output
IBR = insect bite reaction
IC = intracellular (inside the cell)
ICD = irritant contact dermatitis
ICS = intercostal space
ICU = intensive care unit
ID = infectious disease/identification
IDDM = insulin dependent diabetes mellitus
IEC = intradermal carcinoma
If = inflammation
IfR = inflammatory response / reaction
IG/Ig = immunoglobulin
IHSS = idiopathic hypertrophic subaortic stenosis
IL = interleukins = immunoglobulins = Ab
IM/im = intramuscular
IMV = intermittent mandatory ventilation
In = infection
INF = intravenous nutritional fluid
IPPB = intermittent positive pressure breathing
IR = immune response / reaction
IRBBB = incomplete right bundle branch block
IRDM = insulin resistant diabetes mellitus
IT = intrathecal
ITP = idiopathic thrombocytopenic purpura
IV/iv = intravenous
IVC = intravenous cholangiogram/inferior vena cava
IVP = intravenous pyelogram
Ix = investigation of
Iy = injury

J

JN = junctional naevus
JODM = juvenile onset diabetes mellitus
jt(s) = joints = articulations
JVD = jugular venous distention

K

KA = keratocanthoma
KOR = keep open rate
KP = keratous pilaris
KUB = kidneys, ureters, bladder
KVO = keep vein open

L

L = left / lumbar
l = lymphatic
LAD = left axis deviation/left anterior descending
LAE = left atrial enlargement
LAHB = left anterior hemi-block
LAP = left atrial pressure or leukocyte alkaline phosphatase
LBBB = left bundle branch block
LDH = lactate dehydrogenase
LE = lupus erythematosus
lig = ligament
LIH = left inguinal hernia
LK = lichinoid keratosis
LL = lower limb
LLL = left lower lobe
LM = light microscopy
LMM = lentigo maligna (melanoma)
LMP = last menstrual period
LNMP = last normal menstrual period
LOC = loss of consciousness/level of consciousness
LP = lumbar puncture / lichen planus / Low power / lumbar plexus
Lt. = Latin

M

M = margin (generally of the skin)
m = muscle
MAO = monoamine oxidase
MAP = mean arterial pressure
MAST = medical anti-shock trousers
MBT = maternal blood type
MC = metacarpal
MCH = mean cell haemoglobin
MCHC = mean cell haemoglobin concentration
MCL = mid clavicular line
MCTD = mixed connective tissue disease
MCV = mean cell volume
med. = medial
MI = myocardial infarction/mitral insufficiency
mL/ml = millilitre
MLE = midline episiotomy
MM = malignant melanoma / mucous membrane
MM = malignanat melanoma
MMEF = maximal mid expiratory flow
Mmol = millimole
MMR = measles, mumps, rubella
MNC = mononuclear cells
MO = microorganisms
MRI = magnetic resonance imaging
MRSA = methicillin resistant staph aureus
MP = medium power
MS = multiple sclerosis/mitral stenosis/morphine sulphate
MSSA = methicillin-sensitive staph aureus
MT = metatarsal
MVA = motor vehicle accident
MVI = multivitamin injection
MVV = maximum voluntary ventilation

N

N (s) = nerve(s)
NA = nucleic acids
NAD = normal (size, shape) / no active disease/ no abnormality detected
NAD = no active disease/ no abnormality detected
NAS = no added salt
NCV = nerve conduction velocity
NED = no evidence of recurrent disease
Ng = nanogram
NG = nasogastric
NIDDM = non-insulin dependent diabetes mellitus
NK = natural killer
NKA = no known allergies
NKDA = no known drug allergies
NMR = nuclear magnetic resonance
NMSC = non-melanotic skin cancer
NNT = need to treat
nocte = at night
NPO = nothing by mouth /nil by mouth
NR = nerve root origin
NRM = no regular medications
NS = nervous supply / nerve system
NSAID = non-steroidal anti-inflammatory drugs
NS = nervous system
NSR = normal sinus rhythm
NT = nervous tissue / nasotracheal

O

O = origin
OB = obstetrics
OCG = oral cholecystogram
OD = overdose / right eye
OE / O/E = on examination
OM = otitis media
OOB = out of bed
OP = out patients - hospital patients treated but not admitted
OPV = oral polio vaccine
OR = operating room
OS = left eye
OU = both eyes

P

P = para / pressure
PA = posteroanterior
PAC = premature atrial contraction
PAD = peripheral vascular disease
PAO2 = alveolar oxygen
PaO2 = peripheral arterial oxygen content
PAP = pulmonary artery pressure
PaNS. = parasympathetic nervous system
ParaNs = parasympathetic nerves ± fibres
PAS = periodic acid Schiff's stain
PAT = paroxysmal atrial tachycardia
P&PD = percussion and postural drainage
Pb = prothrombin time / lead
PC = after eating
PCWP = pulmonary capillary wedge pressure
PD = pathological diagnosis
PDA = patent ductus arteriosus
PDR = physicians desk reference
PDx = provisional diagnosis
PE = pulmonary embolus /physical exam / pleural effusion
PEEP = positive end expiratory pressure
PFT = pulmonary function tests
Pg/pg = pictogram
ph = palanges
PHx = past history
PI = pulmonic insufficiency disease / pulmonary index
PKU = phenylketonuria
pl. = plural
PMH = previous medical history
PMI = point of maximal impulse
PMN = polymorphonuclear leukocyte (neutrophil, polymorph)
PN = peripheral nerve
PND = paroxysmal nocturnal dyspnea
PNS = peripheral nervous system
polymorphs = polymorphonuclear leukocyte (neutrophil)
post. = posterior
PPD = pigmented purpuric dermatosis
PR = petechial rash
prn = given as required no set treatment regime
proc. = process
prox. = proximal
PS = pubic symphysis / pulmonic stenosis
PT = prothrombin time, or physical therapy

P *continued*

Pt = patient
PTCA = percutaneous transluminal coronary angioplasty
PTH = parathyroid hormone
PTHC = percutanous transhepatic cholangiogram
PTT = partial thromboplastin time
PUD = peptic ulcer disease
PUPP = puritic urticarial papules and plaques of pregnancy
PVC = premature ventricular contraction
PVD = peripheral vascular disease

Q

q = every (e.g. q6h = every 6 hours)
qd = every day
qh = every hour q4h, q6h.... every 4 hours, every 6 hours etc.
qid = four times a day
QNS = quantity not sufficient
Qod = every other day
Qs/Qt = shunt fraction
Qt = total cardiac output

R

R = right / resistance
RA = rheumatoid arthritis or right atrium
RAD = right atrial axis deviation
RAE = right atrial enlargement
RAP = right atrial pressure
RBBB = right bundle branch block
RBC = red blood cell
RBP = retinol-binding protein
RBS = random blood sugar
RBT = random breath test
RDA = recommended daily allowance
RDW = red cell distribution width
RE = rectal examination
RIA = radioimmunoassay
RIH = right inguinal hernia
RLL = right lower lobe
RLQ = right lower quadrant
RML = right middle lobe
RNA = ribonucleic acid
R/O = rule out
ROM = range of motion
ROS = review of systems
RPG = retrograde pyelogram
RRR = regular rate and rhythm
RT = respiratory therapy / radiation therapy / Respiratory tract
RTA = renal tubular acidosis
RTC = return to clinic
RU = resin uptake
RUG = retrograde urethogram
RUL = right upper lobe
RUQ = right upper quadrant
RV = residual volume
RVH = right ventricular hyperthrophy
Rx = treatment / regime

S

S = strata/stratum /sacral
s = without
SA = sinoatrial
SAA = synthetic amino acid
S&E = sugar and acetone
SBE = subacute bacterial endocarditis
SBFT = small bowel follow through
SBS = short bowel syndrome
SC = spinal cord / subcutaneously
sc = subcutaneously
SCC = squamous cell carcinoma
SCr = serum creatinine
SEB K = seborraeic keratosis
SEM = systolic ejection murmur
SG = Swan-Ganz (catheter)
SGA = small for gestational age
SGGT = serum gamma-glutamyl transpeptidase
SGOT = serum glutamic-oxaloacetic transaminase
SGPT = serum glutamic-pyruvic transaminase
SIADH = syndrome of inappropriate antidiuretic hormone
Sig = write on label
SIMV = synchronous intermittent mandatory ventilation
sing. = singular
SK = solar keratosis
sl = sublingual
SLE = systemic lupus erythematous
SMO = slips made out
SN = spinal nerve
SO = standing orders
SOAP = Subjective, Objective, Assessment, Plan
SOB = shortness of breath
SP = spinous process / sacral plexus
SPF = sun protection factor
SQ = subcutaneous
SS = signs and symptoms
ss = one-half/same side/signs & symptoms
SSM = superficial spreading melanoma
SSMM = superficial spreading malignant melanoma
STAT = immediately
STD = sexually transmitted disease
subcut. = subcutaneous (just under the skin)
sup. = superior
supf. = superficial
SVD = spontaneous vaginal delivery
Sx = symptoms
SyNS = sympathetic nervous system

T

T = TEST / thoracic / tissue
T&C = type and cross
TAH = total abdominal hysterectomy
T&H = type & hold (blood or serum products)
TB = tuberculosis
TBG = total binding globulin
TCR = T cell receptor
Td = tetanus-diphtheria toxoid
tds = three times daily
TIA = transient ischemic attack
TIBC = total iron binding capacity
Tid/td = three times a day
TIG = tetanus immune globulin
TKO = to keep open
TLC = total lung capacity
TMJ = temporo-mandibular joint
TNF = tumour necrosis factor
TNTC = too numerous to count
TO = telephone order
TOPV = trivalent oral polio vaccine
TPN = total parenteral nutrition
TS = thin sections
TSH = thyroid stimulating hormone
TT = thrombin time
TTP = thrombotic thrombocytopenic purpura
TU = tuberculin units / transurethral
TUR = transurethral resection
TURBT = TUR bladder tumors
TURP = transurethral resection of prostate
TV = tidal volume
TVH = total vaginal hysterectomy
Tw = twice a week
Tx = therapy / treatment / transplant

U

UA = urinalysis
UAC = uric acid /umbilical artery catheter
UAO = upper airway obstruction
UBD = universal blood donor
UC = ulcerative colitis /umbilical cord
Ud = as directed
UFH = unfractionated heparin
UGI = upper gastrointestinal
UL = upper limb, arm
URI = upper respiratory infection
URQ = upper right quadrant
URTI = upper respiratory tract infection
US = ultrasound
UTI = urinary tract infection
UUN = urinary urea nitrogen
UVA = ultraviolet A light

V

V = vertebra / vein
v = very
VA = verrica / verrucous
VAD = venous access device
VB = vertebral body
VC = vertebral column/ vital capacity
VC = vital capacity
VCT = venous clotting time
VCUG = voiding cysourethrogram
VDRL = Venereal Disease Research Laboratory (test for syphilis)
VE = vaginal examination
VMA = vanillymadelic acid
VO = verbal order / voice order
V/Q = ventilation - perfusion
VRE = vancomycin-resistant enterococcus
VSS = vital signs stable
VT = ventricular tachycardia
VV = varicose veins
vv = visa versa
VW = vessel wall
VWD = von Willebrand's disease
VZV = varicella zoster virus

W

WB = whole blood
WBC = white blood cell / white blood cell count
WBR = whole body radiation
WD = well developed
WF = white female
WIA = wounded in action
WID = widow, widower
WM = white male
WN = well nourished
w/n = within
w/o = without
WNL = within normal limits
WO = written order / weeks old / wide open
WOP = without pain
WOS = wedge of skin
W.P. = whirlpool
WPW = Wolff-Parkinson-White (syndrome)
W-T-D = wet to dry
W/U = workup

X

X2d = times 2 days.
XI = eleven
XII = twelve
XL = extended release / extra large.
XM = crossmatch
XMM = xeromammography
XOM = extraocular movements
XRT = X-ray therapy (radiation therapy)
XS = excessive
XULN = times upper limit of normal

Y

y = years / yes
YF = yellow fever
YLC = youngest living child
yo = years old
YOB = year of birth
yr = year
ytd = year to date

Z

ZDV = zidovudine
ZE = Zollinger-Ellison (syndrome)
Z-ESR = zeta erythrocyte sedimentation rate
Zn = zinc
ZnO = zinc oxide
ZSB = zero stools since birth
& = and
∩ = intersection with
= fracture / number
~ = approximately
º = no (e.g. FFFTº = no fits, faints or funny turns)
1º = primary
2º = secondary
9/12 = nine months
3/52 = three weeks
5/7 = five days
2/24 = two hours
3/60 = three minutes
3/360 = three seconds
3s = three seconds

Extra abbreviations...

Common Histological Stains and their uses

Histology stains are a confusion of eponymous terms and methods used in individual laboratories. In many cases individual variations exist in different laboratories and it is advised that contact with the appropriate laboratory will give the medical professional the details they need, concerning their particular specialities and variations on these common stains. Those included here are those stains common to most labs and the principles behind the staining methods. There are many more and this list is by no means complete, also one stain may be used for many purposes eg the routine stain used in all labs. - H&E. More details can be found in the A to Z of Histology/Histopathology, and the A to Z of the Skin and surface anatomy.

General Stains

Haematoxylin and Eosin (H&E)

This is an all round stain and used on nearly every section in the histology laboratory. The haematoxylin stains the nucleic acids and other acid material blue and the eosin acts as a counter stain to colour most other structures non-specifically red/pink, allowing an overall view of the cellular morphology. It generally does not interfere with other stains and can be used in conjunction with them, for example with PAS.

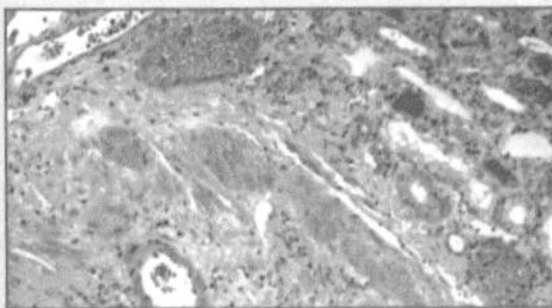
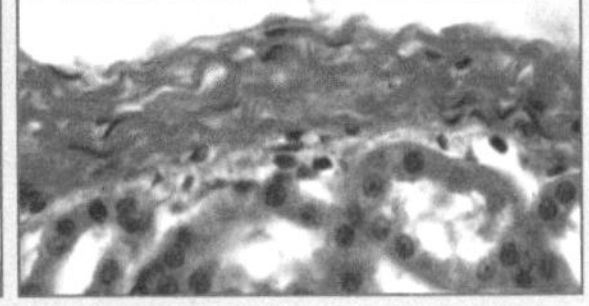

Kidney tissue LP & HP to show clarity of the H&E stain – arrow pointing to the renal capsule with collagen fibres – eosin staining and nuclei of the renal tubules – haematoxylin staining.

PAS (periodic acid-Schiff)

This is an all-around useful stain for many things: glycogen, mucin, mucoprotein, glycoprotein, as well as fungi.
A predigestion step with amylase will remove the glycogen and reduce the background. PAS is useful for outlining tissue structures: basement membranes (BM), capsules, BVs, etc. It is very sensitive, but not very specific.

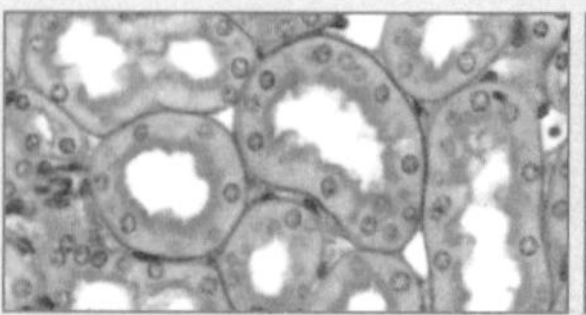
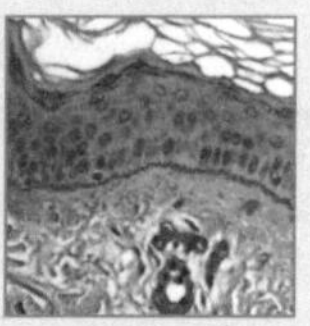

Skin (MP) and kidney tissue (HP) stained with PAS to demonstrate the BM counterstained with H&E.

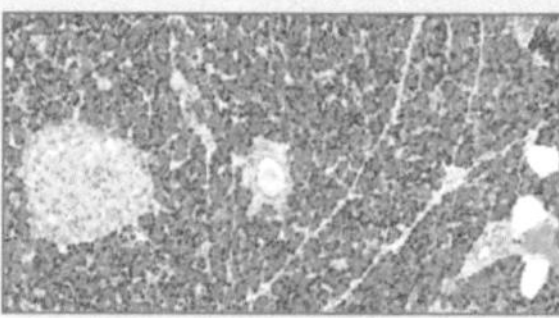
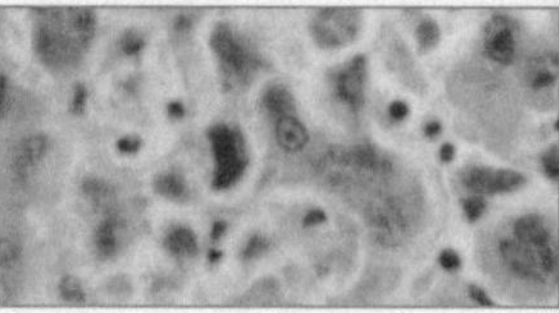

Pancreas (LP) stained with PAS to differentiate b/n the Islets of Langerhans (endocrine) (1) and the glands for digestion containing mucopolysaccharides – PAS +ve (2).

Liver (HP) stained with PAS which stains glycoproteins but also lipofuscin while bile and haemosiderin which do not stain also appear brownish, so structures are unable to be differentiated.

Structures stained

AFB (acid fast bacilli) stain for mycobacterium

This stain uses carbol-fuchsin to **stain the lipid walls of acid fast organisms such as *M. tuberculosis*.** The most commonly used method is the Ziehl-Neelsen method, though there is also Putt's stain, Kinyoun's method a modification of which is the Fite-Faraco stain and has a weaker acid for supposedly more delicate ***M. leprae* bacilli.** Lipid is often removed in the processing, so this stain can be insensitive particularly when looking in large granulomatous tissue. The most sensitive stain for mycobacteria is the Auramine-Rhodamine stain which requires a fluorescence microscope for viewing. There are things other than mycobacteria that are "acid fast". Included are *cryptosporidium, isospora,* and the hooklets of *cysticerci.*

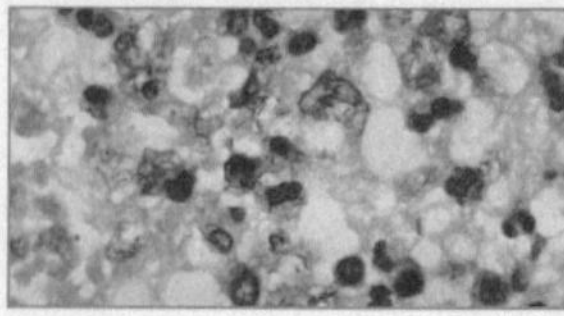

Lung tissue +ve for TB (HP) showing mycobacterium - Ziehl-Neelsen - acid fast stain small purple rods in the cells are the bacteria.

Amyloid

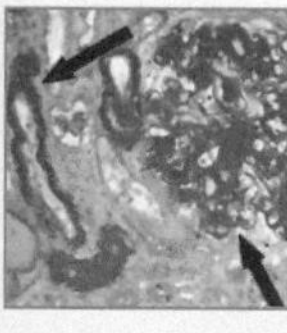

Amyloid is a substance which can be found in all tissues pathologically. Although a fatty substance it is not fat, but can be stained using Congo red, or Lieb's Crystal Violet method, although not with PAS.

Renal tissue showing amyloid in the tubules and glomeruli with Crystal Violet.

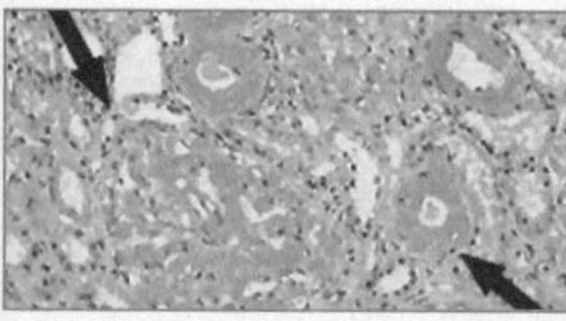

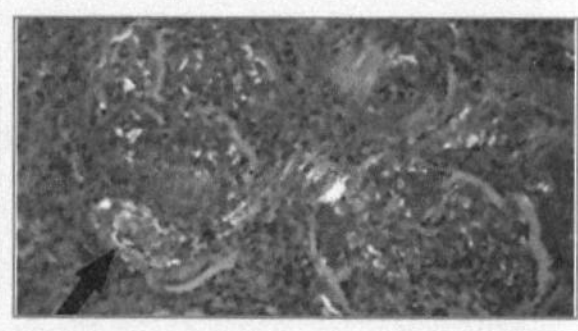

Amyloid in the same tissue stained with Congo red – also showing the apple green birefringence when viewed under polarized light.

Biogenic Amine stains for Argentaffin cells

(Autofluorescence, Diazo, Fontana-Masson, modified Giemsa, Schmorl's Pascual's and Weisel's stains)

Cells that produce polypeptide hormones, active amines, or amine precursors (adrenalin = epinephrine, noradrenalin = norepinephrine) can be found individually (Kulchitsky cell of GI tract) or as a group (adrenal medulla). The following is a traditional classification of the staining patterns based upon the ability of the cells to reduce soluble silver nitrate to metallic silver - causing a black deposit in tissue sections.

Traditionally there are 3 patterns of staining although this is fairly artificial, as they are interchangeable when the fixative is changed. **Chromaffin** cells have cytoplasmic granules that appear brown when fixed with a dichromate solution as in the adrenal medulla and their tumours pheochromocytomas; **Argentaffin** cells reduce a silver solution to metallic silver after formalin fixation, as in carcinoid tumours of the gut. Using a pre-reduction step may cause a more intense stain. This is called an **argyrophil** (silver loving) reaction.

Blood smear stains

Romanowsky stains eg Giemsa stains, Wright-Giemsa stains

All these stains contain mixtures of methylene blue, azure, and

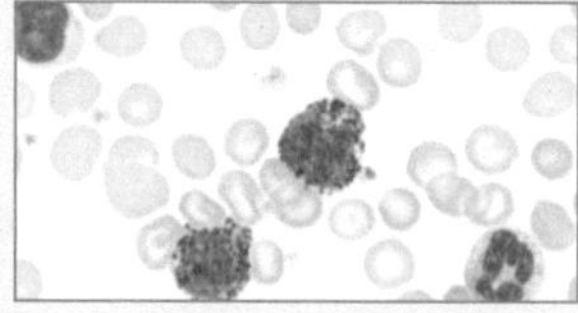

Typical blood smear (HP) showing monocytes (m) and granulocytes - basophils (b) and neutrophils (n) using the one stain - Romanowsky

eosin compounds. One property of methylene blue and toluidine blue dyes is metachromasia. This means that a tissue component stains a different colour than the dye itself. For example, mast cell granules, cartilage, mucin, and amyloid will stain purple and not blue, which is helpful in identifying these components, while using only the one stain.

Calcium (Ca) Stains

Ca bound to an anion, such as phosphate (PO_4) or carbonate (CO_3) can be demonstrated with the Von Kossa stain. Ca forms a blue-black lake with haematoxylin to give a blue colour on H&E stain, usually with sharp edges. This stain is most useful when large amounts are present, as in bone.

Alizarin red S forms an orange-red lake with Ca. It works best with small amounts of Ca (such as in Michaelis-Gutman bodies). The Alizarin method is also used in analyzers to measure serum calcium photometrically.

Azan stain can be used to differentiate osteoid from mineralized bone.

Connective tissue stains (collagen, elastin, reticulin fibres and fibrin)

The trichrome stain helps to highlight the supporting **collagenous stroma** in sections from a variety of organs. This helps to determine the pattern of tissue injury. Trichrome will also aid in identifying normal structures, such as **connective tissue capsules of organs, the lamina propria of gastrointestinal tract, and the broncho-vascular structures in lung**. Sirius red stain is also used for **collagen** staining.

The reticulin stain is useful in parenchymal organs such as liver and spleen to outline the architecture. Delicate **reticular fibres,** which are argyrophilic, can be seen. A reticulin stain occasionally helps to highlight the growth pattern of neoplasms, by showing the dispersal of the normal fibrous architecture.

An **elastic tissue** stain such as the Verhoff's van Giesen stain or Orcein-Giemsa stain help to outline arteries, because the **elastic lamina of muscular arteries, and the media of the aorta, contain elastic fibres**, and if used with the Masson stain for **collagen and muscle fibres** provides a good contrast.

Martius's scarlet blue stain distinguishes **fibrin** from true connective tissues and should be used where there is extensive inflammation.

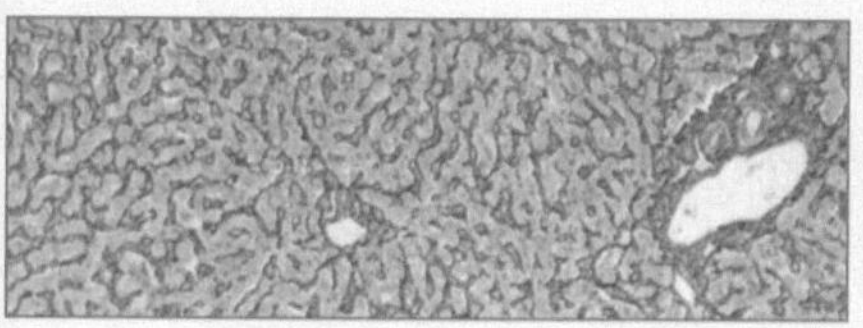
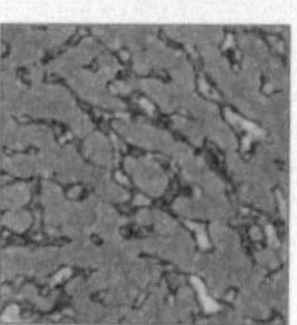

Liver LP and MP stained to show reticular fibres (Gordon & Sweet method) - fine outline of supportive fibres.

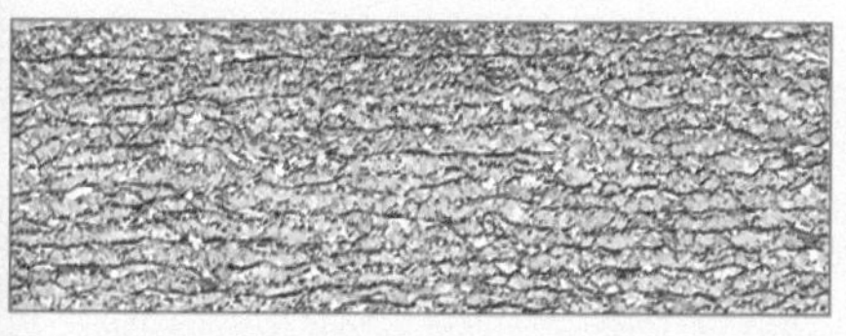

Normal aorta (MP) showing elastic fibres throughout - van Giesen stain.

Exogenous pigments and minerals (asbestos, carbon, silica)

Asbestos is a special type of long-thin silica crystal, usually of the mineral group chrysotile. In tissue, these crystals are highly irritative and highly fibrogenic. The fibres become coated with a protein-iron-calcium matrix, giving them a shish-kebab appearance. These are called "ferruginous bodies" because they are highlighted with an iron stain, such as Perl's iron stain, or the Prussian blue reaction.

Carbon appears as anthracotic pigment in the lungs. It can be distinguished from melanin by doing a Melanin bleach, which helps to distinguish carbon from melanin. Poorly fixed tissues may contain formalin-heme pigment, which is black and finely granular, but this is widely scattered in the tissues without regard to cellular detail. Formalin-heme pigment is also birefringent on polarization.

Silica is present in many minerals and building materials. Most forms are very inert and cannot be stained in tissue but can be demonstrated by white birefringence on polarization. It is most often present in lung, but can make its way into lymph node.

Street drugs for injection often are diluted with compounds containing minerals such as **silica or talc.** These crystals can be found throughout the body, but especially in lymphoreticular tissues. **Tattoo pigment** is usually black and is inert and non-polarizable. **Red tattoo pigment** often contains **cinnabar** (which has mercury in it). There are no specific stains for these materials, and in general, minerals are best demonstrated by microincineration techniques or by scanning electron microscopy with energy dispersive analysis (SEM-EDA), which is also used in the analysis of gunshot residue, because of its composition of antimony, barium, and lead.

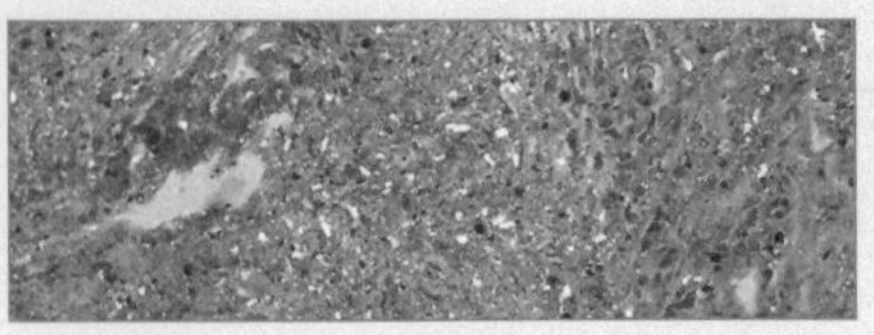

Lung tissue LP in birefringent light to show silica particles in silicosis.

Fat stains

The oil red O (ORO) stain can identify neutral lipids and fatty acids in smears and tissues. Fresh smears or cryostat sections of tissue are necessary because fixatives containing alcohols, or routine tissue processing with clearing, will remove lipids. The ORO is a rapid and simple stain. It can be useful in identifying **fat emboli in lung tissue or clot sections of peripheral blood.**

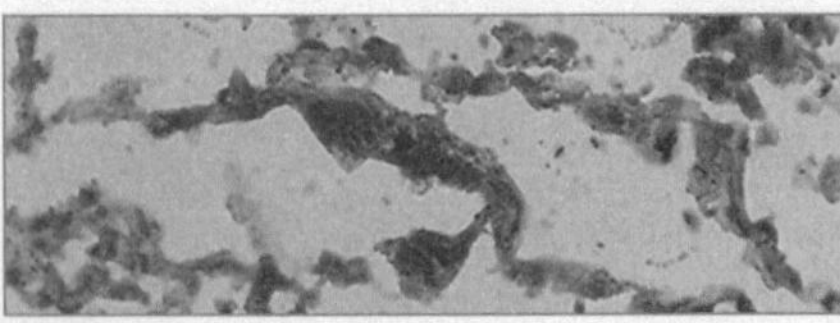

Lung tissue showing fat emboli stained red with Oil red stain (MP).

Fungi stains

(Gomori methenamine silver stain = GMS)

Fungi and *Pneumocystis carinii.*, have cell walls which stain black or brown, outlining the organisms clearly. A disadvantage of this stain is the large amount of background staining, so the morphology of the organism needs to be known. Fungi also stains red with the PAS method and blue with H&E.

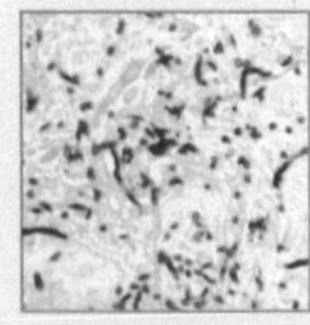

Lung tissue MP stained using the Gomori method to show Aspergillus fungi (a) as long black rods - there is also a background of carbon particles (also black- c) and hard to distinguish except on shape.

Iron (haemosiderin) stains

Haemosiderin (storage iron granules) may be present in areas of old haemorrhage or be deposited in tissues with iron overload (haemosiderosis - physiological, haemochromatosis - pathological).

Perl's iron stain is the classic method for demonstrating iron in tissues. The section is treated with dilute hydrochloric acid to release ferric ions from binding proteins. These ions then react with potassium ferrocyanide to produce an insoluble blue compound (the Prussian blue reaction).

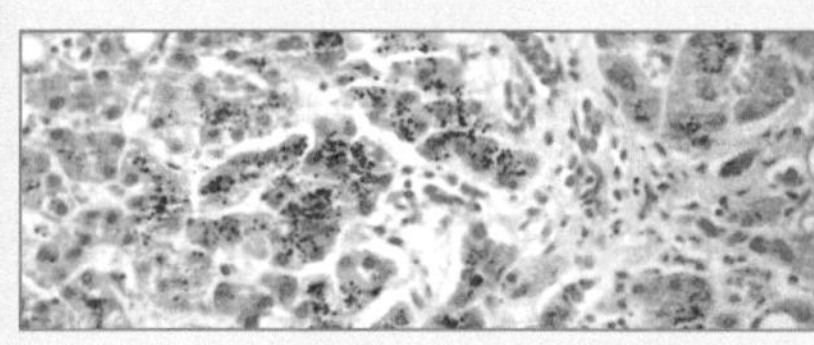

Cirrhotic liver (MP) stained with Perl's stain to demonstrate haemosiderin which contains iron (blue granules).

Lipochrome (lipofuschin) pigments - Age spots

These are the breakdown products within cells from oxidation of **lipids and lipoproteins.** They are the wear-and-tear pigments found most commonly in heart, liver, CNS, and adrenal cortex (zona reticularis). The less highly oxidized "ceroid" pigment of testis interstitium and seminal vesicle is another form of lipochrome.

Lipochrome can be stained by Sudan black B, long Ziehl-Neelson acid fast, and Schmorl's methods. **Lipochrome** may also exhibit a strong orange autofluorescence in formalin-fixed, unstained paraffin sections.

Melanin stains

The Fontana-Masson stain, relies upon the **melanin granules** to reduce silver nitrate (note, argentaffin, chromaffin, and some lipochrome pigments will stain black as well). Schmorl's method uses the reducing properties of **melanin** to stain granules blue-green, but the most specific method is an enzyme histochemical method, DOPA-oxidase. DOPA substrate is acted upon by DOPA-oxidase in the **melanin-producing cells** to produce a brownish black deposit.

Bleaching techniques remove **melanin** in order to get a good look at cellular morphology. They make use of a strong oxidizing agent such as potassium permanganate or hydrogen peroxide. **Ocular melanin** takes hours to bleach, while **skin melanin** takes minutes. Formaldehyde-induced fluorescence can be used to highlight biogenic amines (chromaffin, argentaffin) and melanin in tissues. Formalin fixation imparts a strong yellow autofluorescence to unstained tissues with these substances. **Pseudomelanin** of melanosis coli is PAS positive whereas true melanin is not. **Pseudomelanin pigment** is also found in **macrophages.**

Microorganisms - bacteria stains

Gram stain. Gram positive organisms stain purple and gram negative organisms stain red poorly. In H&E all bacteria appear as blue rods or cocci regardless of gram reaction. Colonies appear as fuzzy blue clusters. **Spirochetes** are very difficult to stain. The best method is the Warthin-Starry stain. A Giemsa stain may help demonstrate **Donovan bodies and leishmania**.

Mucin stains

There are a variety of mucin stains, all attempting to demonstrate one or more types of mucopolysaccharide substances in tissues. The types of **mucopolysaccharides** are as follows:

- Neutral - glands of the GI tract and in prostate. They stain with PAS.
- Acid (simple, or non-sulphated) - are in epithelial cells containing sialic acid. They stain with PAS, Alcian blue, colloidal iron method, and metachromatic dyes.
- Acid (simple, mesenchymal) found in tissue stroma and sarcomas - These contain hyaluronic acid. They stain with Alcian blue, colloidal iron, and metachromatic dyes.
- Acid (complex, or sulphated, epithelial) - These are found in adenocarcinomas. PAS, Alcian blue, colloidal iron, mucicarmine, and metachromatic stains are positive.
- Acid (complex, connective tissue) - found in tissue stroma, cartilage, and bone and include substances such as chondroitin sulphate or keratin sulphate. They stain with Alcian blue.

There are a variety of stains for **mucin:**

- Colloidal iron ("AMP") - stain acid mucopolysaccharides.
- Alcian blue - stains all mucins using a variety of methods
- PAS (peroidic acid-Schiff) - stains glycogen as well as mucins
- Mucicarmine - specifically stains epithelial mucins.

The mucin stain with the most specificity is mucicarmine, but it is very insensitive. PAS is most sensitive but least specific. Colloidal iron stains are unpredictable. Alcian blue stains are simple, but have a lot of background staining.

Urates

Uric acid crystals are seen in acid urine. In tissue, urates are present as **sodium urate.** They are soluble in aqueous solutions and slightly soluble in weak alcoholic solutions. Therefore, tissues must be fixed in 95% or absolute alcohol to prevent leaching of urates. Methenamine silver stains urates black. Sodium urate crystals are also birefringent on polarization.

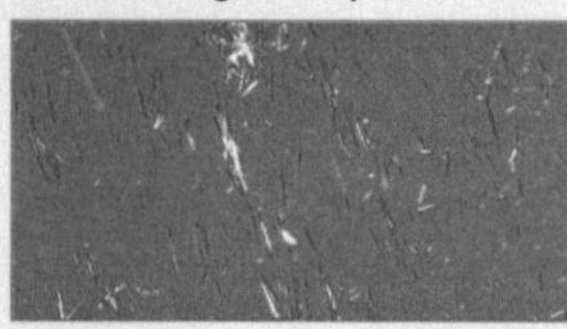

Birefringent urate crystals.

Common Exogenous materials found in tissues

substance	usual site	origin
aluminium	lungs, skin	air / mining
asbestos	lungs	air / asbestos building materials / mining
beryllium	lungs, skin	mining
carbon	lungs, skin	gas emissions, traffic, smoking
fungal spores	lungs, skin, hair	mould, fungi, gardens
lead	kidney, bone, lungs, mucosal linings	paint, mining
silica	lungs, skin	glass, fibreglass material
silver	nasal passages, respiratory mucosa, skin	photography materials, silver, mining

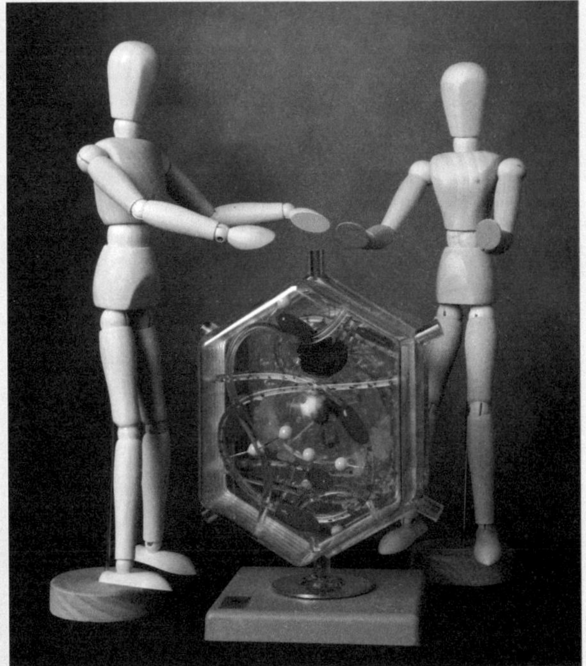

Dimensions in Histology

Based on one metre (m). 1mm (millimetre) = 10^{-3}m
1μm (micrometre) = 10^{-6}m; (nanometre) = 10^{-9}m; 1pm (picometre) = 10^{-12}m

Logarithmic scale of microscope dimensions

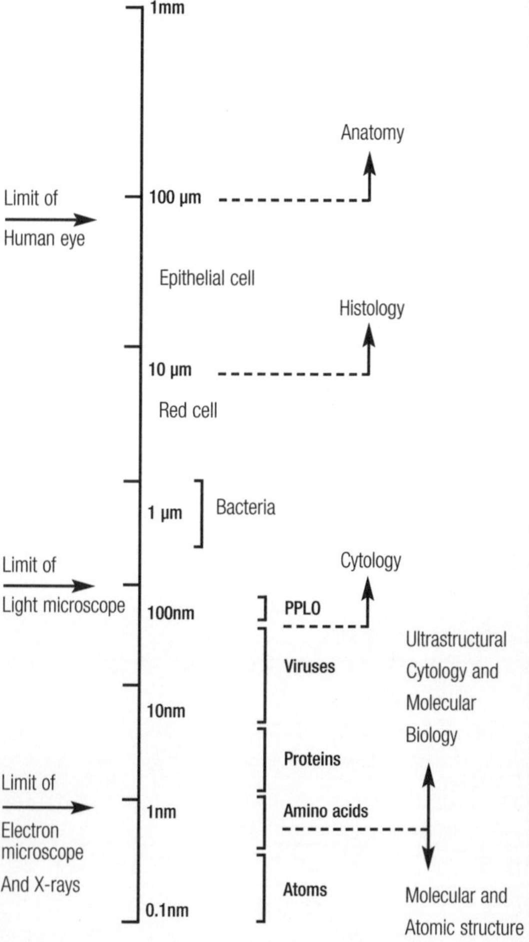

How to Use the Pronunciation Guide.

Words are written in **Bold** with a (bracketed guide) listed afterwards in English sounds - the syllables in CAPITALS are the syllables emphasized in the pronunciation of the word.

Words with a guide are often listed twice the pronunciation guide is first and the etymology or derivation of the word is then listed next with further explanation if necessary.

Please note spelling is both English and American with cross reference to each.

These are the sounds represented in this guide:

a-c*a*t
b-*b*ed
d-*d*og
e-g*e*t
f-*f*at
g-*g*et
h-*h*it
j-*j*og
k-*k*it
l-*l*eg
m-*m*en
n-*n*et
o-g*o*t
p-*p*et
r-*r*at
s-*s*at
t-*t*op
u-m*u*g
v-*v*an
w-*w*in
x-fo*x*
y-*y*et
z-*z*oo

air-*air*
ang-s*ang*
ar-c*ar*
ay-d*ay*
ch-*ch*at
ee-s*ee*
eh-d*ir*t
ehl-b*ell*
er-s*ir*
eye-sk*y*
ing-s*ing*
kew-*que*
oe-b*oo*k
oh-g*o*
ong-l*ong*
oo-d*o*
or-m*ore*
oy-j*oy*
ow-n*ow*
sh-*sh*e
th-*th*e
ung-s*ung*
ya-*yu*k
yew-*you*
uh-li*a*r

Summary of prefixes, word roots and suffixes

Prefixes	Word root	Suffixes
A-: without / no	abdomin- abdomin, belly	-ac / -aceous: pertaining to
Ab-: away from	acanth- spiny, thorny	-acousia: condition of hearing
Ac-/Ad-: towards / near	acar- mite, itch	-ac: state or quality of
Acu-: sharp / sudden	acet- vinegar	-ad: towards
	acetab- saucer	
	acou- hearing	
	acr- extremities	
	actin- ray	
	aden- gland	-adeni: state of glands
	adenoid- glandlike	
	adip- fat	
Af-/ Ag-: near / going to	aemia- blood	-aemia /-emia: blood
	aer- air	-aethesia /-esthesia: condition involving sensation
	aesthesi- feeling, perception	-adol: an analgesic
	aeti- cause	-age: rate action or process
	ala- wing	-agnosia: loss of ability to know
Alb-: white	alg-/ algesi- pain	-agra: pain or painful seizure

Prefixes	Word roots	Suffixes
All-: other different	aliment- nourishment	-al: pertaining to
Ambi-: both	alveoli- air sac	-ance /-ancy: quality or state
Ambly-: dull	amm- sand	-algesia /-algia: sensitivity to pain
Ametri-: disproportionate	amnio- with foetal membranes	-arche: beginning
Amphi-: both sides, both, double	amyl- starch	-ary: pertaining to
An-: without / lack of	andr- man	
	angi- blood vessel	
Anis-: unequal / dissimilar	an- anus, anal	
Anomalo-: unequal, abnormal	anth- floral	
Ante-: before	anthrop- man, human	
Anti-: against	antr- antrum, sinus	
Anykl-: bent, crooked, looped	aqua- water	
	argyr- silver	
	arrhen- man, male	
	artereo- artery	
	arthr- joint	
Apo-: away from, detached	articul- joint surface	
	aster-, astr- star	-aster: star shaped
Asthen-: weakness	ather- fat	-asthenia: weakness
At-: towards	atm- gas, atmosphere	-ate: to use / act like / subject to
Atel-: imperfect	atri- waiting room	-atresia: condition of occlusion

Prefixes	Word root	Suffixes
Atreto-: imperfect / imperforate, closed	audi- hearing	-atrophia: condition of malnutrition / wasting
Auto-: self	aur- ear, ear shape	-aux /-auxe: enlargement
Aux-: growth, increase	auri- gold	
	axi- axis, axial	
	axilla- armpit	
	azot- nitrogen, urea	
Ball-: throw	balan- glans penis	
Bar-: pressure	bar- pressure, weight	-biosis /-biotic: life
Basi-: base, foundation	blenn- mucus	-blast: bud forming / immature / embryonic
Bi-/ Bin-/ Bis-: two	blephar- eyelid	-blepharia: re the eyelid
Brachy-/ Brevi-: short	brachi- arm / upper arm / gill	-blepsia /-blepsy: condition of sight
Brady-: slow	branchi- gill	-brachia: to do with the arm
	bronchi- air transport in the lung / branch	-bund: prone to
	bucc- cheek	
Cac-: diseased, abnormal	calc- heel / lime /calcium	-cace: bad / diseased / deformed
	calor- heat	
	canth- slit for eyelids	
	capill- small tube or hair	

	capit-/ caput- head	
Cat-/ Cath-: down / against	caps- capsule	
	carcin- cancer of epithelial origin	
	cardi-/ cardio- heart	-carcinoma: cancer of the epithelial cells
	carp-/ karp- wrist	-cardia: to do with the heart
	cary-/ kary- nucleus	-cathartic: cleaning
	case- cheeselike	
	caus-/ caut- burn / burning	
	caud- tail	
	caul- stem	
	cav- cavity, hole, hollow	
Cen-/ Coen-: general	cel-/ coel- cavity / something coming through a hole e.g, a hernia	
		-cele /-coele: hernia, tumor or swelling / cavity of the body
	centr- central	-centesis: puncture
	cephal- head	-centric: with a centre
	cer- wax	-cephalia: to do with the head
	cerat- cornea/ horny tissue	-cerebral: pertaining to the brain
	cerebell- little brain	-chesia: pertaining to faeces defecation
	cerebr- brain	

Prefixes	Word root	Suffixes
	cervic-, cervix- neck	
	chal- copper	-cerebral: pertaining to the brain
	chancr- rotting, growing abnormally, cancer	-chesia /chezia: to do with defecation
	cheil-/ chil- lip	-chondria: condition of worrying about a disease
	cheir / chir- hand	-chromasia: condition of colour
	chol- bile / gall bladder	
	chondro- cartilage	
	chord- cord, string	
	chrom- coloured	
	chron- time	
	chyle- digested food / fats	
	cili- eyelash / eyelid	-chylia: condition of digestion
Circum-: around, circular / surrounding	cilia- hairlike / hair	-cide: to kill killer
Cirrho-: yellow	cine- movement	
Cis-: on this side / on the same side	clast- breaking / an instrument which breaks	
Cleist- /Clist-: closed	cleid- clavicle	-clasia /-clasis /-clast /-clastic: crushing or breaking up
	clin- to bend	-cle: little diminutive
Co-/ Col-/ Com- / Con- /Cor-: together with	col-/ coel- colon	-cleisis: closure, conclusion

Contra-: against	colp-/ kolp- vagina	-clonia: re spasms
	con-/ kon- dust / together, with	-cnemia: condition of leg below the knee
	cor-/ coron- heart / crown	-coccus: berry shaped
	core- pupil	-comma: a piece of something
	corp- body	-crania: re the head
Cryo-: cold	cost- rib	-crasia: a condition of / a mixture
Crypto-: hidden	crani- skull	-cratia: re incontinence
Cyano-: blue	cresc- to grow / to expand	-crine: secretion eg glandular
	crur- leg	-cule /- culum /-culus: diminutive
	cusp- point	-current: running, flowing
	cutis- skin	-cusis: hearing
	cycl- circle /cyclical	-cyst /-cystic: bladder / fluid filled sac
	cry-/ kry- frost	-cyte: cell / mature cell
	cyst- bladder / sac of fluid	-cythemia / cythaemia: condition of cells of the blood
	cyt- cell	
De-/ Des-/ Dis-: remove, undo	dacry- tears	
Demi-: half	dactyl- fingers / toes	-dactyl: condition of fingers or toes
	dem- people	-demic: relating to a region
	dent-/ dont-/ odont- tooth, toothlike, teeth	-dendron: treelike formation

Prefixes	Word root	Suffixes
	der- neck	-dermia: skin
Dextra-: right	derm-/ dermato- skin	-desis: binding / fixation
	desm- bond / bind / ligament	-desma: bridging or connecting
Di-: two	digit- finger / toe	-dipsia: thirst
Dia-: through / between / apart	dors- back	-dontia: to do with teeth
Diplo-: double / twin		-drome: that which follows a specific path
Dis-/ Dys-: difficult / wrong / incorrect		-dynamia /-dynamy: strength, power
Duo-/ Dy-: two	dur- hard	-dynia: condition of pain
E-/Ec- / Ecto: outside / external		
Ectro-: absence / congenital	echin- spikey	-eal: pertaining to
Ef-: move away / go away / outside	ec- house	-ectasia /-ectasis /-ectasy: expansion, stretching
Em-/ en-/ endo-: within inside	ele-/ eole- oil	-ectomy: excision of / cutting out
Ent-: inner within	emet- vomiting	-ectopia: out of place
Ep-/ epi-: upon, in addition to, over	encephalo- brain	-edema / oedema: swelling
Equi-: equal	entero- gut / intestine / GIT	-eidos: shape, form
Eryth-: red	episi- vulva	-ellum: small, diminutive
Eso-: within, inside	erg- work / activity	-emetic: pertaining to vomit
		-enchyma: nourishing of cells and structures

	ergy- action	-eous: composed of / like
	erot- love desire	-ergetic/-ergic: effect of activity
Eu-: normal, well		-ergy: effect or result
Ex-/ exo-/ extro-: external, outside, protruding		-escent: become like / emitting light
Extra-: in addition to		-esis: action / process or the result of
	faci- face	-fast: securely attached confined
	fasci- band or sheet (of CT)	-febrile: feverish
	febri- fever	-ferous: bearing
	ferr- iron	-fibroma: benign tumor of fibrous tissue
	fibr- fibrers / to do with fibres	-flect / -flex : to bend
	fila- threadlike	-fluent: to flow
Flav- : yellow	fiss- split / cleft	-form / forme: to have a shape
Fore- : before, in front of	foet-/ fet- to do with foetus	-fuge: to drive away
	for place / opening	
	fract- break	
Fund- : to pour / the body of	fus- spindle	
	galact- milk	
	gam- union	-gamy: marriage, union
	gangli- knot	-gen: that which generates
	gastri- stomach	-genesia: condition concerning information

Prefixes	Word root	Suffixes
	gemin- twin	-genisis: origin
	gen- race /sexual/ reproduction	-genia: condition of the jaw
	geni- chin	-genic: origin , formation
	genu- knee	-geusia / geustia: to do with taste
	geny- under the jaw	-glia : to glue, stick, adhesion
Ges- : to carry, bear	ger-/ geri-/ geront- old / aged	
	gingivi- gum	
	glia- glue / gluelike	-gluten : glue
	gloss-/ glosso- tongue	-glossia: to do with the tongue
	glyc- sweet / sugar	-glycaemia: condition of sugar in the blood
Gravis-: heavy	gnath- jaw	-gnathia: condition of the jaw
Gymno-: naked	gn- know / discern	-gnomy: science of judging
	gon-/ knee / sexual /semen	-gnosia: condition of knowing
	goni- corner / angle	-gony: birth origin
	gran- grain-like/ granular	
	gravid- pregnancy	
	gyn/ gyno/ gynaeco- female	-gyne: female characteristics
Hapl-: single	haeme-/ heme- blood	
	hallux- big toe	

PREFIXES, WORD ROOTS, SUFFIXES

Prefixes	Word roots	Suffixes
Hemi-: half	hel- horn /corn	
Hetero-: different	helc- ulcer, sore	
Holo-: entire, whole	heli- sun	
Homo-/ Homeo-: same / level	helic- spiral	
Hyper-: excessive	hepat- liver	
Hypo-: less than normal	hidr-/ hidro- sweat	
	hier- sacrum	-hydat : water
	hist/ histo- tissue	-hydria: fluid level in the body
	horm- to stimulate	
	hyal- glasslike, glassy	
	hydr- water, wet / hydrogen	
	hyster -uterus	
Il- : negative, against		
Im-/ In- : in, into / onto/ no, non	iatro- to treat	-iatric: to treat / cure
Infra-: below , beneath / inside	icter- jaundice	-iatrician: physician / healer
Inter- : between	ide- mind	-iatry: specific type of medical condition
Intra- : within	idi- distinct / separate	-ible: ability, capacity
	ili- pertaining to the flank or lower abdomen	-ic /ical/: pertaining to / similar to
	ima- below, beneath, the lowest inguin- groin	-id: state or condition, structural element of teeth

PREFIXES, WORD ROOTS, SUFFIXES

Prefixes	Word root	Suffixes
	ini- back of the head	-ism: resulting from practice or theory of
Ithy- : straight	insul- island	-ismus: spasm / contraction
	irid- iris of the eye, rainbow colours	-ist: agent, person, practitioner
	isch- suppression / stoppage	-itic: relating to
	ischi- hip	-itis: inflammation of
		-ium: diminutive
	jug- yoke	
	jugu- throat / neck	
Juxt-: next to	juxta- next to	-kine stimulation/activation of cell division or growth
	kali- potassium	-kinesia: condition relating to movement
	kaps- capsule	-kinesis: division of cells / activation
	kary-/ cary- nucleus	
	kerato- horny	
Koilo-: hollow / concave	kinesi- movement	
	kolp-/colp- vagina	
	labi- lip	-labial: pertaining to the lips
Laevo-/ levo-: left	lac- milk	-labile: unstable, changeable
Leio-/ lio-: smooth	lacri- tears	

Lep-: to take or seize	lal- talk / babble	-lalia: condition involving speech
Lepto-: thin, narrow / small	lamina- layer, veneer	-lemma: sheath, envelope / confining membrane
	lapar- abdominal cavity	
	lapis- stone	
	laryng- voice box / voice	
Leuco-/ Leuko/ Luco-/ Luko-: white/		
colourless/ pale	lat/later- side	-lepsis /-lepsy /-leptic: seizure
	lex- read	-lexia: reading conditions
	lien- spleen	
	lim- hunger	
Liga- bind together	lingu/lingua- tongue/tonguelike	
	lip- fat	-lipsis / lipse: leave / fail / omit
	lith- stone	-lith /lithiasis: stone / re stones
Longus-: long	loc- place	-logia: condition of speech or reason
Loxus-: oblique	luc-/ leuc- light /white/ pale	-logology: study or science of
	lue- syphilis	
	lumb- loin / lower back	-lucent: light admitting
	lumin- light/ cavity / channel	
	luna- moon	-lymph: clear fluid
	lyc- wolf	

Prefixes	Word root	Suffixes
	ly- dissolve	-lyse /-lyze /-lysis: to decompose / to breakdown
	lys- disintegrate	-lytic: production of / decomposition
Macro-/ Makro-: large	malar- cheek bone	-ma/ -mata: result of an action
Magna- : huge	mamm- breast	-malacia: softening
Mal-: bad	man- hand	-mancy: divination
Malac- : soft	mania- obsession	-mania: obsession, compulsion
	mast-/ mastoid-/ maz- breast / breastlike	-manic: specified psychosis
	maxilla- upper jaw	-mastia/ -masty /mazia/: re the breast
Medi-/ Mes-: middle	maz- breast	-megaly: enlargement
Meg-/ Megalo-: large, great	meat- opening /hole	-melia: re the limbs
	mel- cheek / limb / member	-mentia: re the mind
Meio-/ Mio-: reduced, contraction	melan- dark / black	-mere /-mer /meria: part of / condition of the parts
Meli-: sweet/ honey	men- periods, menstruation, menses	
Meta-: extension of subsequent transformation	mening- membrane	-meter: measurement
	menisci- disc / crescent	
	ment- mind / chin	
	mer- part	
	metop- forehead	

PREFIXES, WORD ROOTS, SUFFIXES

	metr- mother, uterus	-metria: re the uterus
Micro-: small	micr- small /abnormally small	-metry: re measuring
Mid-: middle	mit- threadlike	-mimesis: imitation / simulation
Mis-: hatred	mnem- memory	-mittent: send
Multi-: many	morph- form	-mnesia: re the memory
	mot- movement	-moria: condition of dementia
	muc-/myx- mucus	-motor: effects of activity
	my- muscle	
	myc- fungal	
	myel- bone marrow /spinal cord	-myelia: re the spinal cord
	myl- molar	
	myring- eardrum	
	narc- stupor	
	naris- /nas- nose	
Necr-: death	necr- death	
Neo-: new	nephr- kidney	-nephric: re the kidney
	neuro- nerve / brain	-neural: re nerves structurally
	noci- pain	-neuria: a condition of nerves
	nod- knot	

Prefixes	Word root	Suffixes
	nos- disease	
	not- back	
	nucha- neck, nape of neck	
Ob-/ Oc-: against	occipit- back of the head	
	occlus- to close or shut up	
	ocul- eye	
Oes- : inside, internal	odont- teeth	-odontia: treatment of teeth
	odyn- pain, distress	
	oedem-/edem- swelling	-oedema: condition of swelling
Olig-: scant, few	olfact- smell	-oid: resembling / form
	om- shoulder	-ol: oil
	omphal- navel	
	onc- tumor, mass, swelling / bulk / hooked	-oma: mass, tumor, lump, swelling
	onych-/ onyx- nail	
	o-/oo-/ ovi- egg / ovum	-on: unit
	ooph-/ oophor-/othec- ovary	-opia /-opsia /-opy: condition of vision
	ophthalm- eye	-orexia: condition of appetite
	ops-/ opt-/ optic- eyesight	-osis: disease of (generally non-inflammatory)
	orb- sphere	-osmia: sense of smell

	orch-/ orchid- testis	
	or-/ ora- mouth	-otomy: removal of
Ortho-: straight, correct, normal	os- mouth / bone	
	osche- scrotum	
	osm- odour/impulse/osmosis	
	oss-/ osteo- bone	-osteon/-osteum: bone
	ot- ear	-otia /otic: ear
Pachy-: thick	paed-/ ped- child	-pachy: thickening
Paleo-: ancient old		-paedic /-pedic: children
Pali-: repetition recurrence	palat- roof of the mouth	-path :individual; suffering from a disease / individual treating a disease using a system
Pan-: everything	palpebra- eyelid / eyelash	-pathetic: relating to emotions
Par-/ Para-: against / aside / nearby / abnormal	palpit- flutter	
Parvi-: small	papilla- nipple	
Per-: through	part- childbirth	-pathy: disease of / therapy
Peri-: around / surrounding	path- disease	-pede /-ped: number of feet
Perma-: permanent	pect-/ pector- chest, breast. / thorax	-paenia/ -penia: deficiency of
Pero-: stunted	ped-/ pes- foot	-pepsia /-peptic: state of digestion
	petr- stone	-phagia: eating / desire to eat -

Prefixes	Word root	Suffixes
Phan-/ Phas- visible / speak	phac-/ phak- lens	-phasia /-phemia: re speech
Phen-: light, bright	phag-eater, to eat phalan- fingers / toes	-philia /-philic /-phily: love of, affinity with -phobe /-phobia: resisting / avoiding, fearing, dreading
	phall- penis, penile	-phoresis: transmission
	phas- speech	-phoria: tendency to / emotional state / visual axes
Phleg-: inflammation	phleb- vein, veinous	-phragm: separation
	phren- mind	-phrasia: re speech
	physi- natural	-phrenia: re the mind
	pil- hair	-phrenic: re the diaphragm
Plan-: flat	plantar- sole of the foot	-phyisis: growth, growing
		-phyma: lump
Plat-/ platy-: flat/ broad, wide	plas- grow and form	-plakia: patches on membrane
Pleo-: many	pleo- many	-plasia: condition / formation
Pluri-: many more	pleur- walls of the lungs, thorax	-plasty: repair of / involving surgery
Poikilo-: irregular / abnormal	plic- fold ridge	-plegia /-plegic: paralysis
Polio-: grey	pne-/ pneum- breath, air, lungs, gas	-plex /-plexus: network
	pod- foot	-plexia /-plexy: condition resulting from a stroke
	pollex- thumb	-pnea /-pnoea: breathing, re respiration

PREFIXES, WORD ROOTS, SUFFIXES

	poples- posterior part of the knee	-podia: re feet
Poly-: many	pont- bridge	-poeisis: formation / development
Post-: after	por- passage / pore / callus	-pore: passageway
	presby- old	
Prae-: in front of / young	proct- anus, anal / rectum	-proctia: re the anus
Pre-: before	prosop- face	-prosopia: re the face
Presby-: old	psor- to itch	-pterygium: re the conjunctiva
Prim-: first	psych- mind	-ptosis: downward displacement
Pro-: before, in front of	pter- wing / feather	
	ptoma- corpse	
Pronus-: face down	ptyal- saliva	-ptysis: spitting
Pseudo-: false	ptysis- to cough or spit	
	pub- adult	-pubic: frontal part of the pelvis
	puer-/ pueb- child/infantile / undeveloped	-pulsion: push
Quad-: four	pulm- lung	
	pur-/ py-/ pyron- pus,	-pyrexia: re fever
	pyel- renal pelvis / kidney	
	rachi- spine	
	radi- radiation, ray	-rehexis: break, burst
	radi-/ radicul- roo t/ tooth / nerve	

Prefixes	Word root	Suffixes
Re-: return / again / contrary	rami- branch	
Retro-: behind / go back	rect- rectal / straight	-rrhagia /-rhagia: excessive flow / rupture
Rhabdo-: striped	ren- kidney	-rrhea /-rrhoea: flow, discharge
Rhod-/ Rub-: red	rhabdo- stick, straight / rod	-rrhaphy: suturing in place
	rhachi- spine, vertebral column	
	rhe- flow	-rrhea: flow
	rhig- stiff / cold	
	rhin- nose / noselike	
	rhiptid- wrinkles	
	rhiz- root	
	rost- beek	
	rot- to turn	
Schiz-: split	sangui- blood	
Scirrho-: hard	sanita- health	
Sclera-: hardening	sapr-/ seps- decaying	-scelia: re legs
Scolio-: twisted	sarc-/ sark- muscle / network / flesh	-sclerosis: hardening
Semi-: half	scaph- boatlike	
Sicc-: dry	scat- faeces, dung	

Sinistro-: left	scel- leg	
Spano-: few / scant	schist- split, fissured / cleft	
	schiz- divided	
	scia-/ skia- shadow	
	scolec- worm	
	scope- examine	
	scyt- skin	
	sect- to cut	-sect: to cut
	sens- perception, feeling	-sepsis: condition of decay
	seps- decay	
	sept- wall / to separate / border	
	sial- saliva	
	sider- iron	
	sin- hollow cavity	
	soma-/ somatic- body	
	somn- sleep	
	spasm- tighten / straighten, cause rigidity	-spasm: involuntary contraction
	sperm-/ spermato- seed	
Spheno-: wedge	sphen- wedge	
Spiro-: coil	sphym- pulse	-sphygmia: condition of the pulse
	spin- spine	

Prefixes	Word root	Suffixes
	spir- breath	
	splanchn- visceral, intestines	
	splen- spleen	
	spod- waste materials	
	spondyl- vertebrae spinal column	
	spongi- sponge	-stage: phase
	squam- scale	-stalsis: contraction of the alimentary canal
	stann- tin	
Sten-: narrow, constricted	stas- standing walking stopped	-stasis: to stand to stop
Ster-: solid	steat-/ steap-/ stear- fat	
Strept-/ Stroph-: twisted	stell- star	
	sterc- faeces	
	stern- shield	
	steth- chest	-stole: condition of organs
	stoma- mouth / opening / covering	-stoma: mouth, opening
	strab- to squint	
	strati- to layer / layers	
	stri- line	
	strum- goiter	
Sub-/ Suf-/ Sup-: under	styl- stake pole	-stophy: to twist, turn

Prefixes	Word roots	Suffixes
Super-/ Supra-: over above	succ- juice	
Supinus-: face up	sud- sweat	
Sy-/ Sym-/ Syn-/ Syl-: together, union	syndesm- connective tissue	-synthesis: formation of
	syring- tube	
	tabe- to waste away	
Tach-/ Tachy-: fast	tact- to touch	-taxia: condition of impairment / an arrangement
Taut-: tight same	taenia-/ tenia- a ribbon / a band	
	tal- ankle	-taxis: movement
	talip- club footed	
	taph- grave	
	tars- eyelid / edge of foot	
	techn- the art of	
Tect-/Teg-: covering	tect- roof	
Tors-: twisted	teg- covering	
	tela- weblike	
	tele/ tel- end / far away	
	temp- time	-thecium: sack, container
	teno-/ tend- rope	-thelium: layer of tissue
	terat- monster	

Prefixes	Word root	Suffixes
	test- testimony, witness / testicles	
	thec- sheath	-therapy: re treatment
	thel- nipple	-thetic: to put, to place
	thely- female	-thymia: re the mind and emotions
	thenar- palm of hand / sole of foot	-trichia: re hair
Thyr-: shield	therap- treatment, cure	
	thix- touch	-tomy /-tome /-tomic: re incisions, cutting
Trachy-: rough	thora- chest	-tonia: re muscle contraction
Trans-: across	thrix- hair	-tresia: perforation
Tricho-: hair	thromb- clot, lump	
Trocho-: round	thym- thymus, mind or spirit	
	top- place / to place	
	tox- poison	
	trachel- neck windpipe	
	tract- draw, drag	
Trop-: turn / change	troph- food / to feed	
	typ- model	
Ultra-: beyond	ul- gums / scar	
	ungu- nail	

Uni-: single, one		
	ur-/ urin-/ uron- urinary tract	
	uter- uterus	
	vas- vessel / duct	-verse: to change
	ven- vein	-vorous: re eating
	venter- belly / hollowed part	
	ventr- front	
	vermi- wormlike	
Volv-: turn	vesic- bladder / blister	
	vir- virus	
	viscer- internal organs	
Xanth-: yellow	vivi- living	
Xero-: dry	xen- different, foreign	
	xiphi- swordlike	
	zyg- yoke / union / pair	-zoite: simple organism
		-zyme: re enzymes

Common organ specimens sent to Pathology Laboratories

Tissue / Organ (Specimen types)	Non-Tumor Pathology	Tumor Pathology
Appendix (appendectomy)	appendicitis mucocele	carcinoid tumor 1° or 2° tumor (rare)
Artery (Bx)	arteritis atheroma aneurysm	chemodectoma (eg. carotid body tumor)
Bladder (Bx / cystectomy)	cystitis diverticulae fistulae tuberculosis schistosomiasis	transitional cell Ca SCC adenocarcinoma
Bone / Bone Marrow (Bx)	osteoporosis osteomalacia osteomyelitis Paget's disease	osteochondroma myeloma metastatic tumor (eg breast, bronchus, thyroid, prostate, kidney)
Breast (Bx / mastectomy)	cysts fibrocytic disease abscess fat necrosis	adenoma fibroadenoma adenocarcinoma Paget's disease of the Nipple
Bronchial (Bx)	inflammation squanous metaplasia	SCC oat cell Ca
Cervix (cone Bx / punch Bx)	inflammation dysplasia (CIN)	SCC SCC CIN genital warts
Colon / Rectum (Bx / colonectomy)	UC Crohn's disease amyloidosis fistulae amoebiasis diverticular disease	adenomatous polyps adenocarcinoma lymphoma polyps
Endometrium (Bx / curettings)	endometritis abnormalities of the menstral cycle hyperplasia	adenocarcinoma sarcomas polyps

Epididymis (Bx)	cysts inflammation tuberculosis	adenocarcinoma
Fallopian tubes (Bx / salpinectomy)	salpingitis ectopic pregnancy endometriosis	adenocarcinoma
Gall bladder (Bx / cholecystecomy)	cholecystitis calculi	adenocarcinoma
Joints / Tendons / Synovial membrane (Bx / curretings)	arthritis crystal synvitis (eg gout)	sarcoma
Kidney (Bx / nephrectomy)	amyloidosis glomerulonephritis pyelonephritis cysts calculi tuberculosis	adenocarcinoma transitional cell Ca - pelvis
Larynx / Vocal Cords (Bx)	laryngeal nodules inflammation	polyps SCC
Liver (Bx / lobectomy)	hepatitis cirrhosis obstructive jaundice sarcoidosis amyloidosis storage disorders	hepatocellular Ca lymphoma 2º tumor (eg. breast, colon, pancreas and stomach)
Lung (Bx / pneumonectomy)	pneumonia	SCC oat cell Ca adenocarcinoma 2º tumor (eg. bone, breast and brain)
Lymph node (Bx / radical removal of LN group)	reaction to inflammation tuberculosis sarcoidosis	Hodgkin's lymphoma / non-Hodgkin's lymphoma 2º tumor (eg. breast, colon, lung, testis)
Muscle (skeletal) (Bx)	myopathies neuropathic atrophy	rhabdomyosarcoma
Nasal mucosa (Bx)	inflammation	mucoepidermoid Ca polyps SCC

Oral cavity (Bx)	cysts (dental) inflammation	polyps salivary gland tumors - adenocarcinomas SCC
Oesophagus (Bx)	oesophagitis strictures ulceration (peptic)	SCC
Ovary (Bx / oophrectomy)	cysts endometriosis	benign and malignant tumors of respective tissues epithelium = mucinous cystadenoma stroma = thecoma germ cells = dermoid cyst, dysgerminoma 2º tumor (eg. stomach)
Pancreas (Bx)	cysts pancreatitis	adenocarcinoma (exocrine) apudomas (endocrine)
Parathyoid gland	hyperplasia	adenoma
Placenta / umbilical cord	malformations infarctions	choriocarcinoma hydatiform mole
Pleura (Bx)	inflammation tuberculosis sarcoidosis	mesothelioma 2º tumor (eg. breast, lungs)
Prostate gland (Bx / prostatectomy)	hyperplasia prostatitis	adenocarcinoma
Salivary gland (Bx)	calculi sialoadenitis	adenolymphoma (Warthin's) mucoepidermoid tumor pleomorphic adenoma
Skin / hairy skin (Bx / punch Bx / curettings / shaves / ellipsoid excision / Mohs sections)	cysts dermatitis reactive changes fungal infections alopecia psoriasis	adenocarcinoma BCC carcinoid tumor CIN - Bowen's disease lymphoma melanoma naevi skin tags / polyps SCC warts

Small intestine (Bx / resection of the small bowel partial or complete)	Crohn's disease coeliac disease diverticulae infarction	adenocarcinoma carcinoid tumor lymphoma
Spleen (Bx / splenectomy)	amyloidosis hypersplenism syndromes thrombocytopenic purpura traumatic rupture	lymphoma leukaemia
Stomach (Bx)	gastritis peptic ulceration	adenocarcinoma leimyoma lymphoma
Testis (Bx / orchidectomy)	hydrocoele orchiditis tuberculosis	lymphoma teratoma
Thyroid (Bx / thyroidectomy)	nodular goitre Hashimoto's thyroiditis thyrotoxic hyperplasia	adenoma adenocarcinoma leiomyoma (fibroid) medullary carcinoma (+ amyloid)
Uterus (Bx / hysterectomy)	abnormal cyclical bleeding adenomyosis endometriosis	leiomyoma (fibroid) adenocarcinoma (of endometrium)
Vulva (Bx / excision)	dysplasia inflammation leukoplakia	SCC CIN warts

The A to Z of Histopathology specimen preparation - common errors

Contamination Artifacts

Specimen – Solution contamination

Preparing a surface for biopsy may result in depositing materials such as iron on the surface and masking the pathology e.g. mucosal surfaces painted with MONSEL's solution (ferric sulphate) to stop clotting - iron is absorbed and any from the specimen is masked, see excessive blue staining with PERLS stain (for iron) on normal surface of cervix (H&E).

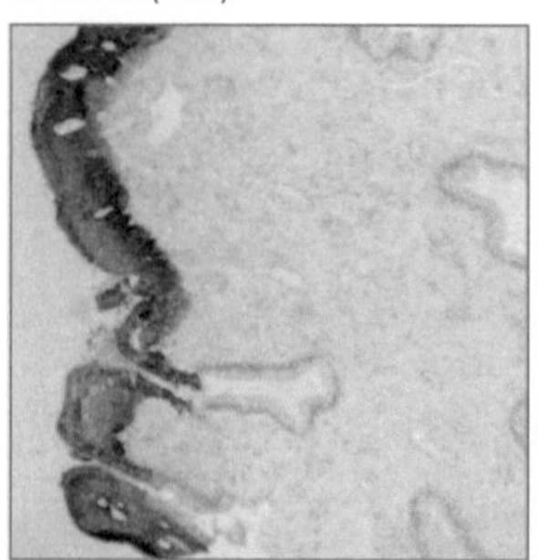

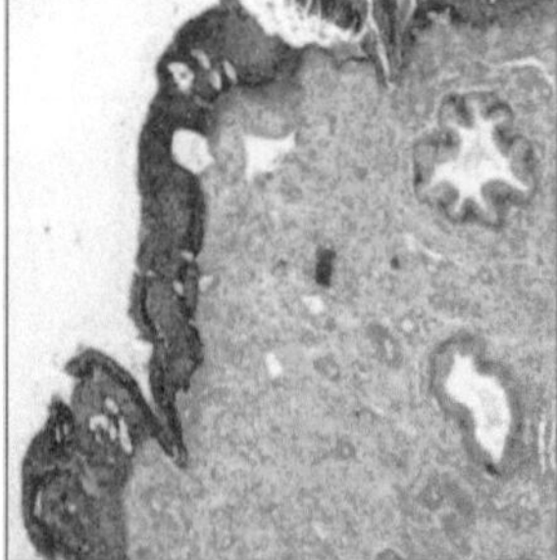

Specimen - Specimen contamination

Taking specimens and not cleaning off the instruments in b/n may result in 2 or more tissues in the one specimen).

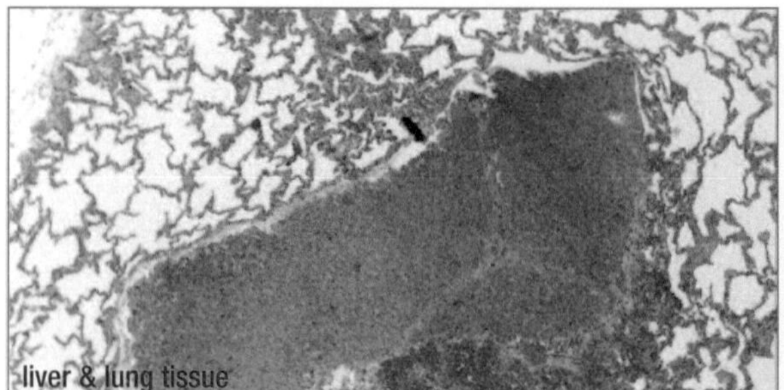
liver & lung tissue

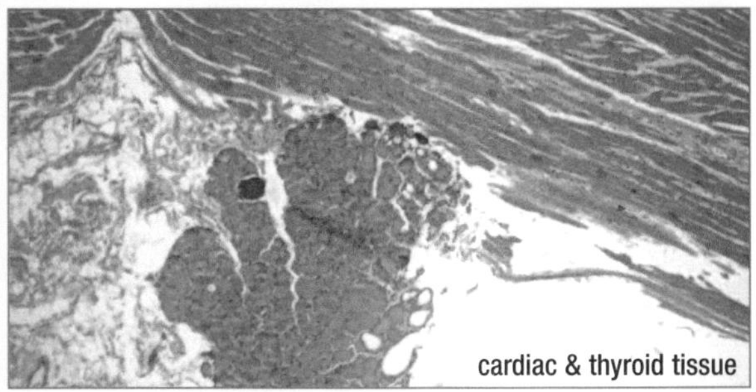
cardiac & thyroid tissue

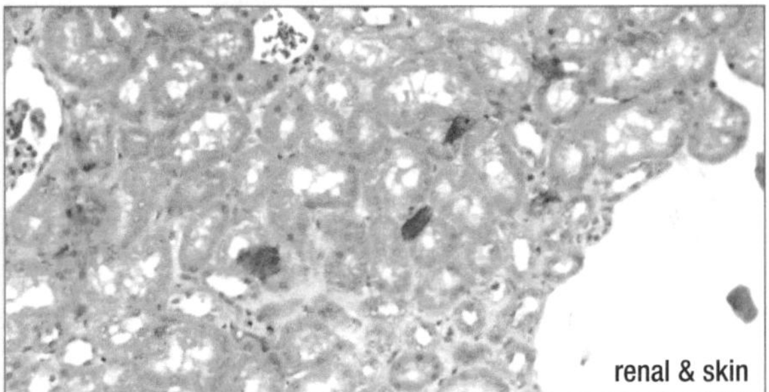
renal & skin

(as floating squamous cells = squames which have come off the hand and attached to the tissue).

Drying Artifacts

Leaving the specimen on the bench particularly on an absorbent surface (filter paper) will dry it and alter the results.

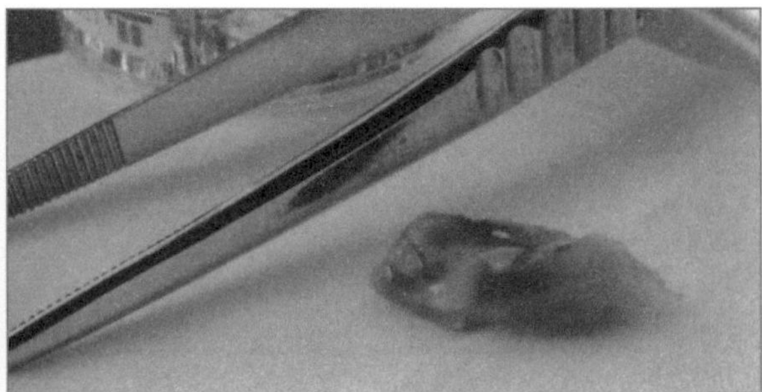

This may cause cracking in the tissue also from other causes such as too much drying on the slide - &/or overprocessing.

Lymphoid tissue overdried showing cracks in the tissue

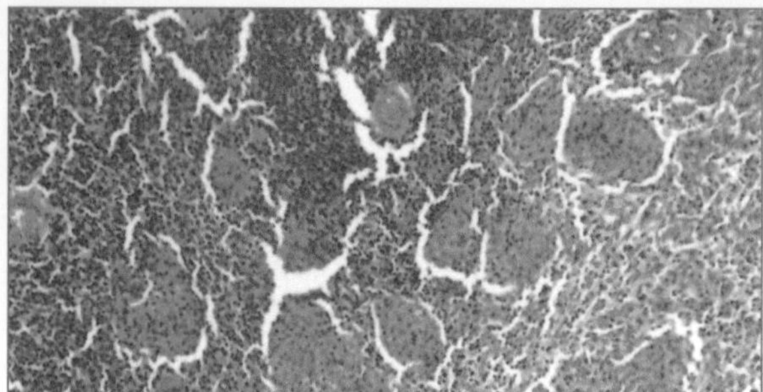

Drying of the surface of the specimen before fixation may result in nuclear staining changes prostate specimen (H&E).

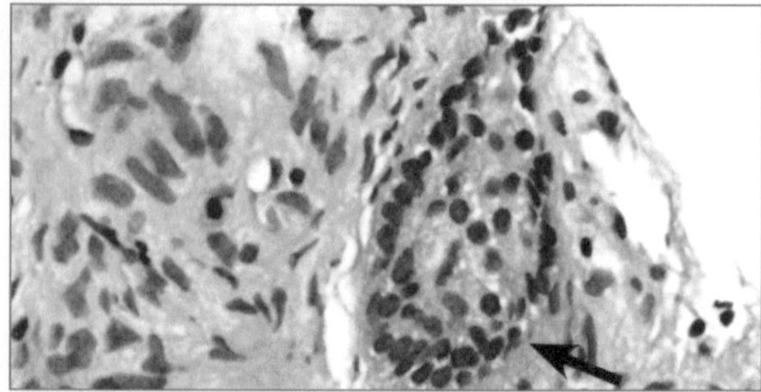

Delaying Artifacts

This is important in frozen specimens or those which need refrigeration or urgent processing.

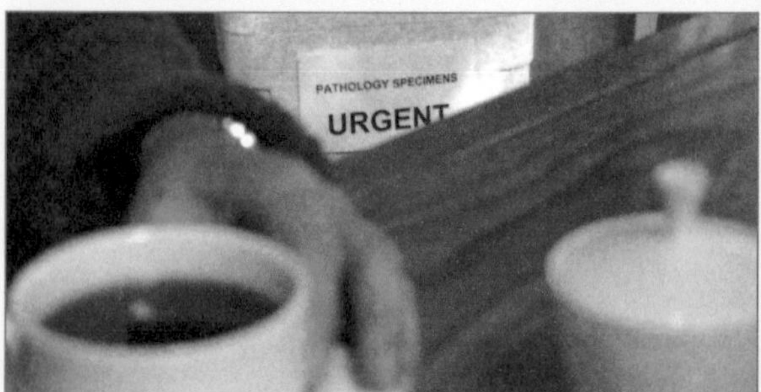

Fixation Artifacts

Fixation / Tissue ratio there should always be minimally 3:1 with the tissue well covered otherwise poor fixative penetration may result.

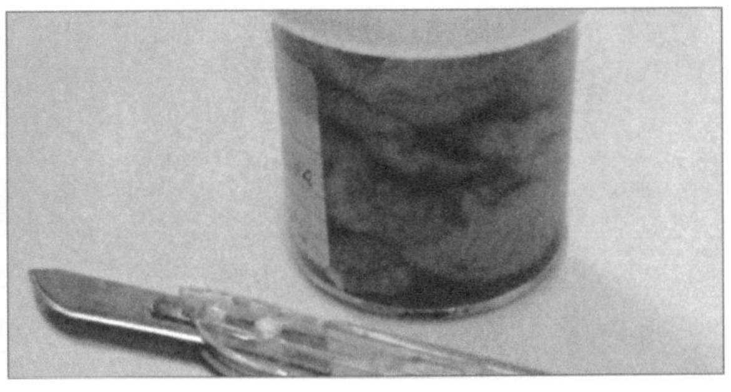

For larger specimens use larger specimen pots and prepare -

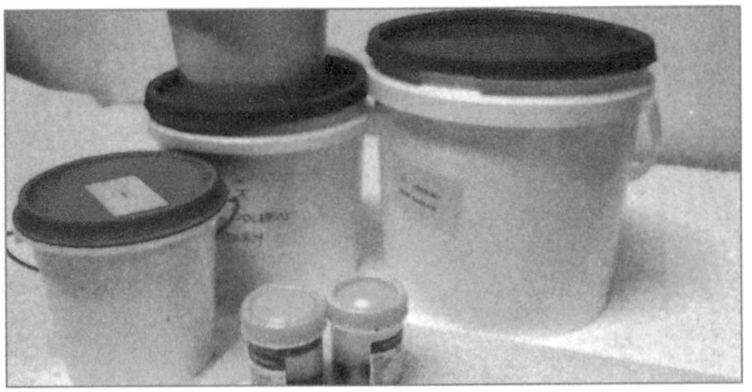

larger specimens with 5-6mm cuts to allow for fixative penetration.

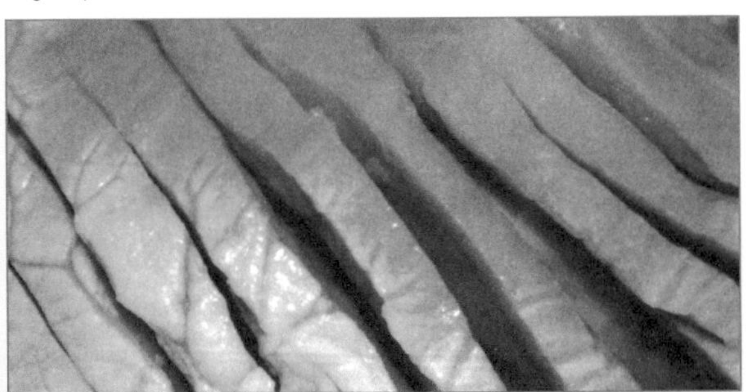

Liver tissue poorly fixed on outer border – no cell definition.

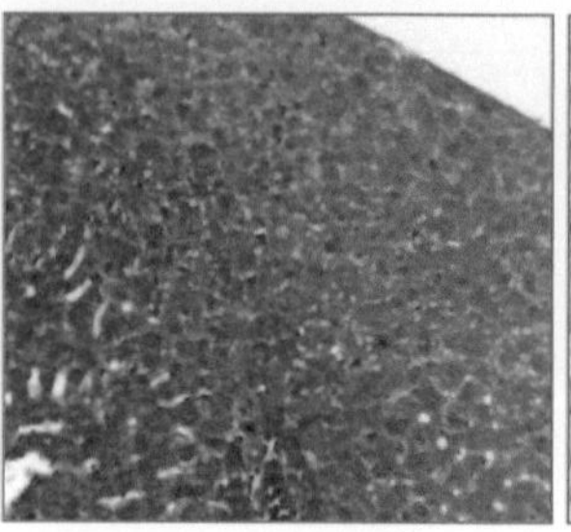

Bone Marrow - no cell definition in the lower edge cannot make out the RBCs

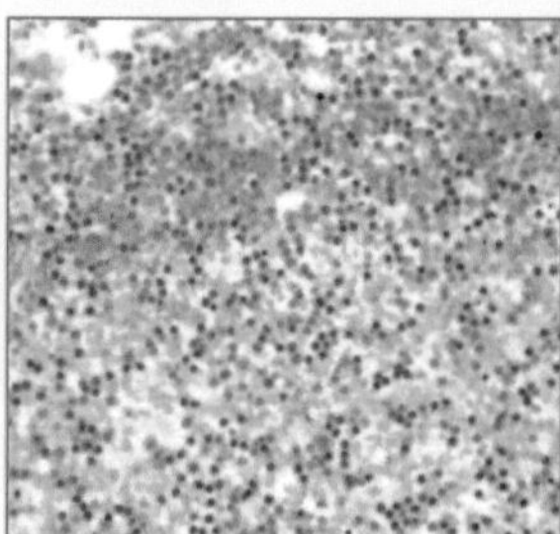

Skin - irregular nuclear staining because of poor inadequate fixation.

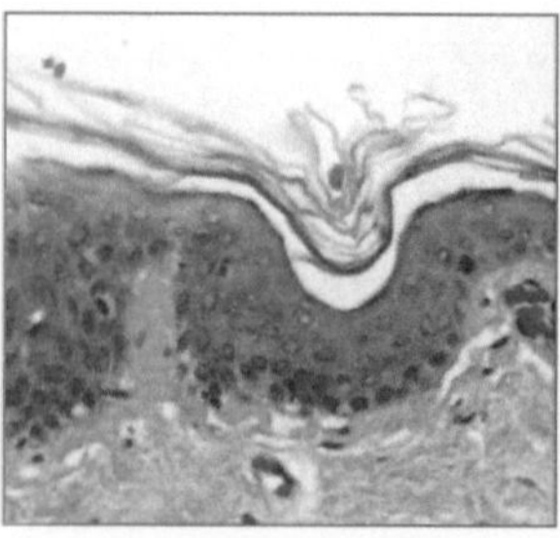

Acidic pH artifact - formalin fixative solution should be 6.8-7.0 if very acidic, deposits can be found in the tissues, particularly in RBCs.

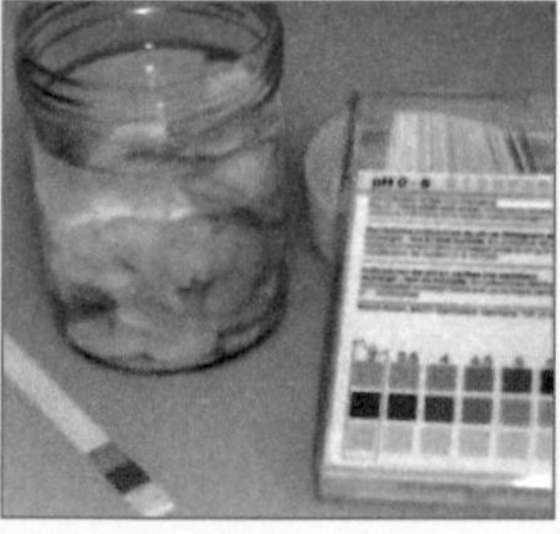

Acidic fixation if not corrected results in haematoxylin not staining the nuclei, as observed in the first image, as opposed to the nuclei normally stained in the second image.

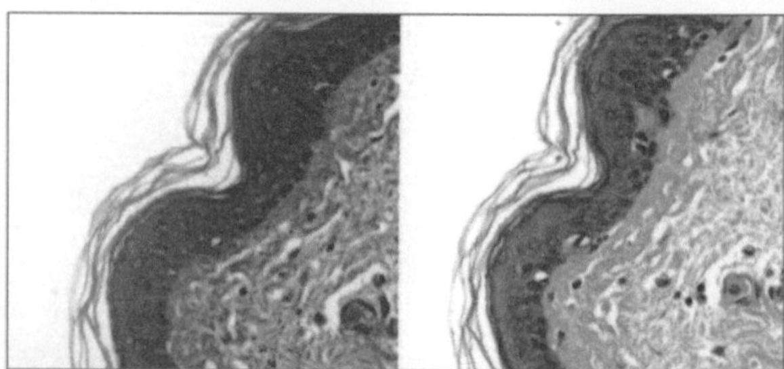

Black deposits in RBCs from formalin acid crystals Alkaline pH artifact – poor eosin staining.

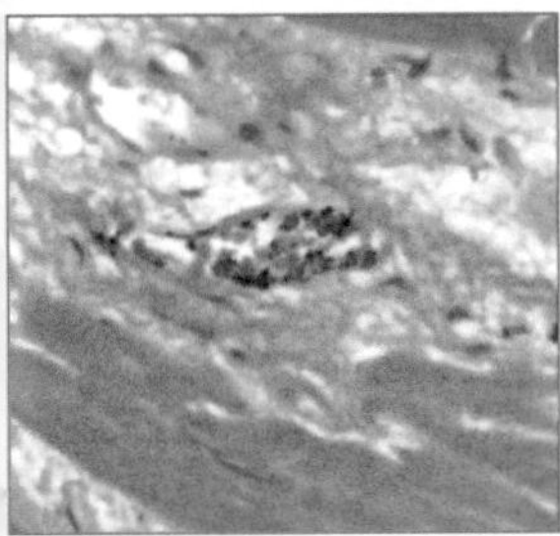

Lung tissue with minimal eosin staining because of high alkalinity.

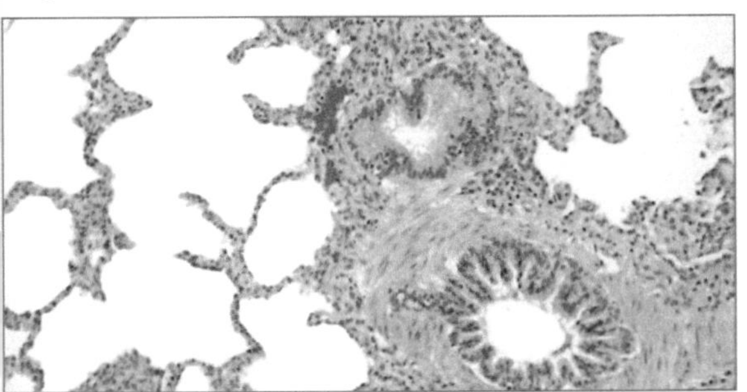

Lymphoid tissue with minimal eosin staining because of high alkalinity.

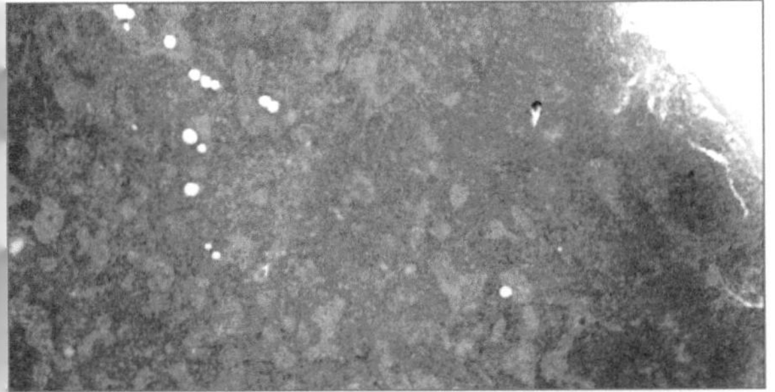

Salivary specimens showing normal glands and abnormal edges hyper-eosinophillic.

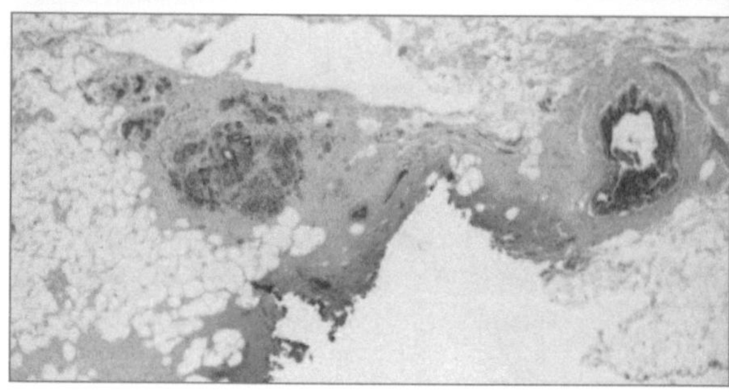

Cracks appearing in **lymphoid tissue** close to heat – also pyknotic nuclei.

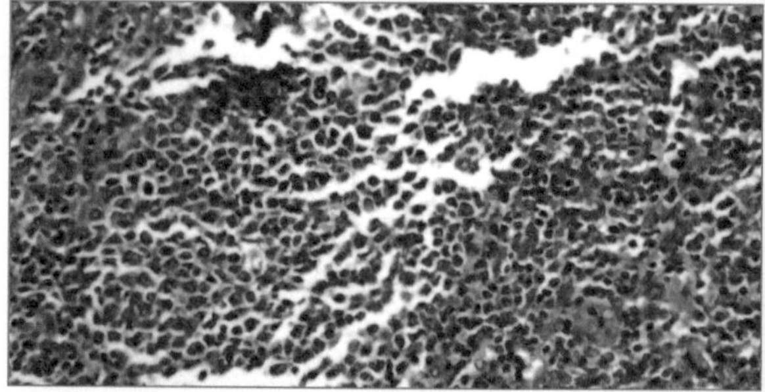

Labelling Artifacts

Insufficient labelling will cause specimen mix up.

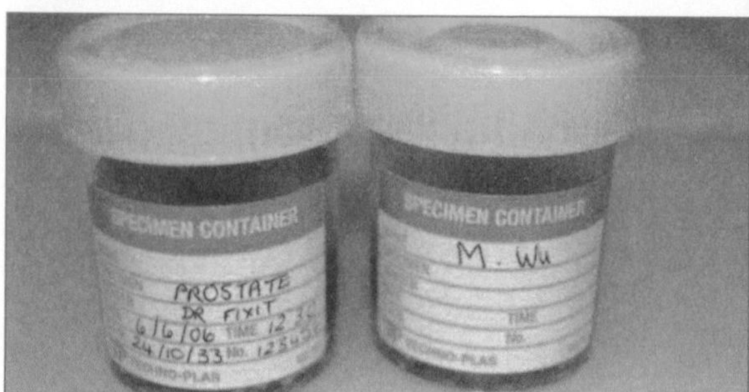

Tissue Trauma Artifacts

Crush injuries – crushing or tearing of the specimen when removing. **Lung tissue** collapsing under trauma.

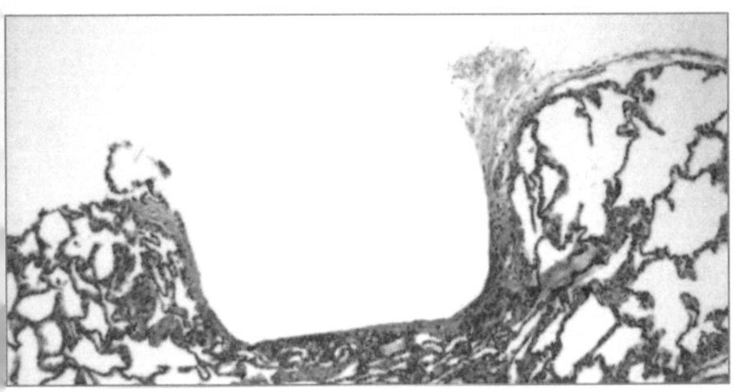

Lymph tissue crushed distorted nuclei because of trauma.

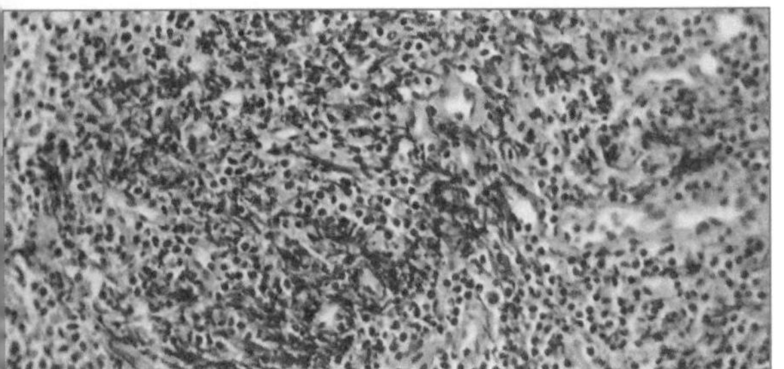

Shake Injuries – shaking of the specimen will result in small pieces breaking off depending upon the tissue's friability. Small pieces break off in the specimen pot – resulting organ architecture cannot be seen. Small pieces may go through the processing cassette and be lost.

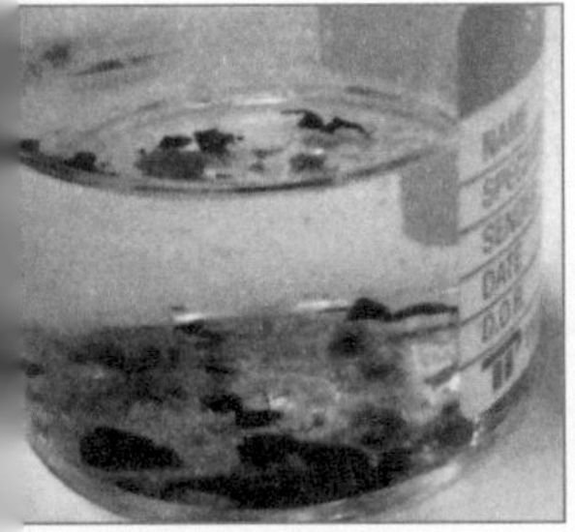

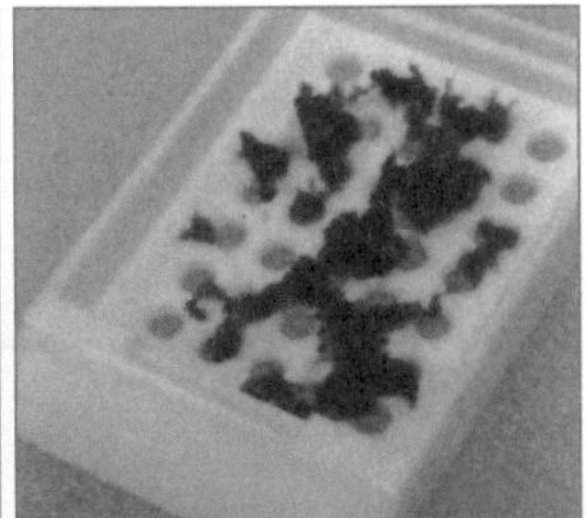

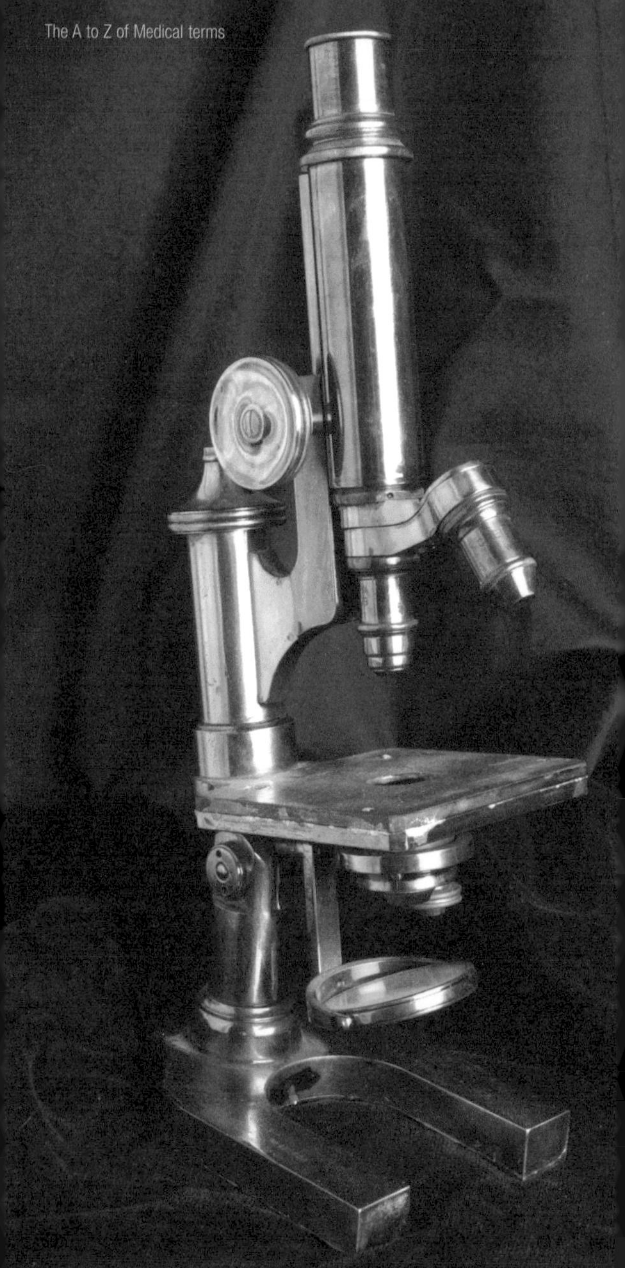

A

a- without, lack of, no
ab- away from, negative
Abcess (AB-sess) localized collection of pus.
 abdomen: Lt. abdomen = the belly, the part of the trunk between thorax and the perineum.
 abduction: Lt. ab = from, and ductum = led, hence, movement from; verb - abduct. (≠adduction).
 aberrant: Lt. ab = from, and errare = to wander, hence, deviating from normal.
Absorption (ahb-SORB-shun) the passage of digested foods from the GIT & into the BS.
ac- toward, near to, addition to
acanth- spiney prickly horny
Acanthosis: (AY-kan-thoh-sis) Gk thorns, prickles - used to describe any thickened skin condition involving the prickle layer Strata Spinosum.
 accessory: adj.Lt. accessum = added, hence, supplementary.
 acetabulum: Lt. acetum = vinegar (cf. acetic), and abulum = small receptacle, a vinegar cup, the socket for the head of the femur, adj.- acetabular.
Achalasia (AY-kal-ay-si-ya) failure of relaxation of smooth muscle.
Acini (AS-ih-nee) clusters of cells in the pancreas that secrete digestive enzymes. sing. acina adj. acinar (AS-in-us).
Achlorhydria (AY-claw-hid-ree-yu) absence of hydrochloric acid in the stomach.
Acne (AK-nee) an inflammatory condition of the pilosebacious unit - hair unit in the skin.
Acoustic (ah-COOS-tic) pertaining to hearing and sounds.
 acoustic: adj.Gk. akoustikos, related to hearing.
acro- extremity
Acromion (AK-croh-mee-on) boney extremity of the shoulder
 acromion: Gk. akros = summit (c.f. Acropolis) and omos = shoulder, the tip of the shoulder.
Actin (AHK-tihn) the contractile protein that makes up the major portion of thin filaments in muscle fibres.
 actin(o)- Gk: actinos – ray
Actinic (AKT-in-ik) related to the sun see also solar.
acou- to hear, pertaining to hearing

A

acu- sudden, sharp, severe

B

Acute (ak-yewt) - sudden onset + short course - used to describe a condition generally pathological ≠ chronic.

C

….acu- Gk: acus = needle.

ad- near, toward

D

additus Lt. = entrance, opening.

E

adduction: Lt. ad = to, and ductum = led, hence, movement. towards; verb - adduct. (≠abduction).

F

aden- gland

G

adenoid: Gk. aden = a gland, eidos = shape or form.

Adenohypophysis: aka = the anterior lobe of the pituitary gland. It is

H

composed of glandular epithelium. The adenohypophysis secretes numerous Hs, several of which affect the activity of other endocrine glands.

I

adhesion: Lt. ad = to, and haesus = stuck.

J

Adipose (AHD-ih-pose) a CT whose cells (adipocytes) are highly specialized for lipid storage.

K

adipose: Lt. adeps = fat, hence fatty.

L

Adnexa (AD-nex-uh) appendage, limb extras pl adnexae (AD- nex-ee)

adrenal: Lt. ad = towards, at, ren = kidney, situated near the

M

kidney (see suprarenal).

N

adrenergic: adj. Gk. ergon = work, stimuli which cause the adrenal (suprarenal) gland to produce adrenaline. A term used to

O

specify neurons or pathways which use adrenaline as a transmitter.

P

Adrenal cortex (ah-DREE-nal KOR-teks) the outer region of the adrenal glands, located superior to each kidney. It secretes steroid

Q

Hs, including glucocorticoids & mineralocorticoids.

R

Adrenal glands two endocrine glands, each situated superior to a kidney, (also = suprarenal glands).

S

Adrenal medulla the inner region of the adrenal glands, which secretes epinephrine and norepinephrine (also adrenaline

T

noradrenalin).

U

Adventitia (ahd'-ven-TISH-yah) the outermost covering of an organ or tissue (see Serosa, Tunica Externa).

V

aero- air, pertaining to gas

W

af- near, toward, addition to

afferent: adj.Lt. af = to, and ferent = carrying (cf. ferry), hence,

X

carrying to, e.g., axons carrying information from retina to lateral geniculate nucleus are afferents to that nucleus.

Y

ag- near, toward, addition to

Z

agger Lt eminence pl aggeres.

agger nasi: Lt. = eminence of the nose - in front of the middle concha.

agglut- (a-GLOOT) to glue

aggreg- to crowd together, to flock.

agno- not to know, inability to know.

agonist: Gk. agonistes = rival, hence, a muscle in apparent contest with another, (a prime mover). adj.- anlagonist.

Ala (AY-lar) referring to the wing or flattened part of a bone particularly if there are other shapes in the bone which are not wide and flat as in the Sphenoid or the inominate / hip.

ala: Lt. wing, hence a wing-like process; pl. - alae.

alaeque: Lt. ala = wing (ala of nose), suffix -que = and, hence levator labii superioris alaeque nasi muscles = lifter of the upper lip and ala of nose.

alb- white

alba: Lt. albus = white.

albicans: Lt. = becoming white; albus = white.

albuginea: Lt. albus = white, Gk. gen = form, like boiled white of an egg.

- algia Gk: algos = pain (AL-jee-uh) -

alimentary: adj.Lt. alimentum = food, e.g., alimentary canal.

alipo- pertaining to fat.

all- other, different, abnormal

allantois: Gk. allantos = sausage, eidos = like, form.

Allergy (AL-er jee) abnormal reaction to a substance.

allo- other, different, abnormal,

Alopecia (AL-oh –peesh-uh) baldness, loss of hair (Gk alopekia = fox mange).

Alpha cell a type of cell in the pancreatic islets of Langerhans that secretes the H glucagon.

alveolus: Lt. a basin, hence any small hollow. pl. - alveoli, adj.- alveolar, after holes in a tissue e.g. the lung - alveolar bone in the maxilla.

Alveolar duct (awl-VEE-o-lar) a branch of a respiratory bronchiole w/n the lungs leading to alveoli & alveolar sacs.

Alveolar sac two or more alveoli which share a common opening from an alveolar duct.

Alveolus (awl-VEE-o-lus); a microscopic air sac within the lungs. pl. - alveoli.

alveolar: Lt. alveus = hollow.

ambi- both, about, around

ambiguus: adj.Lt. = doubtful (nucleus ambiguus).

ambon - the ring of fibrocartilagenous cartilage around the socket of long bone joints.

amin(o) – any organic substance containing nitrogen.

Amnesia (am-NEESH-ya) – loss of memory.

amnesia- Gk = forgetfulness.

amnio- Gk: amnios = bowl - membranes surrounding the foetus (AM-nee-yoh.)

ampulla: Lt. = a two-handed flask, a local dilatation of a tube.

amputation: Lt = amputare to cut off, to prune, to cut off a limb or appendage.

amygdaloid: adj.Gk. amygdala = almond, and eidos = shape or form, amygdaloid is almond-shaped.

amylacea: Gk. amylon = starch, hence, starchy.

amyl(o): Gk amylos = starch, starchlike properties.

Amyloidosis (AM-ill-oy-doh-sis) disease characterized by extracellular depositions of amyloid, a starch-like substance, throughout the body.

an- without, lack of, not

an(a)- up, back, again, excessive

Anaemia (an –EEM-ee-ya) AS Anemia – lack of RBCs or oxygen carrying capacity.

anaemia : GK. an = w/o, aimia blood – lack of blood adj. anaemic

anaesthesia: Gk. an = negative, and aisthesis = sensation, loss of sensation;

Anal canal (A-nawl) the terminal 2 or 3 cm of the rectum. It opens to the exterior at the anus.

analgesia: Gk. an = negative, and algesis = pain, insensibility to pain; adj.- analgesic.

analogous: Gk. ana = up, apart, towards, and logos = word. A part with similar function through different morphology e.g., fish gills and mammalian lungs (c.f. homologous).

Anaphylaxis (AN-uh-fill-ax-sis) exaggerated /unusual reaction to a foreign body = acute allergic reaction.

anastomosis: Gk. ana = of each, and stoma = mouth, hence the end-to-end continuity of 2 vessels.

Anatomical position the reference position, in which the subject is standing erect with the feet facing forward, arms are at the sides, & the palms of the hands are facing forward (the thumbs are to the outside).

Anatomy (ah-NAH-to-mee) the study of the structure of the body.

anatomy: Gk. ana = up, and tome = a cutting, hence cutting up of a body (c.f. dissection).

anconeus: Gk. ancon = elbow, hence the muscle attached to the (lateral surface of the) olecranon.

Aneurysm (an-YOU-ris-sm) pathological widening of an artery.

aneurysm: Gk. angeion = blood vessel (BV), and eurys = wide, a pathological dilatation of a BV.

angina: (ANJ-eye-nuh): Gk angor = a strangling

angio- (ANJ-ee-oh) to do with BVs

angiogenic: Gk angeion: blood vessel, and genic to form, formation of vascular origin.

angiography: Gk. angeion & graphe = a record; picture of a BV injected with radiopaque material.

anhidrosis: (anhydrosis, anidrosis) Gk. an = negative, and hidros = sweat; absence of sweating, typical of skin deprived of its sympathetic innervation.

ankle: the region between the leg and the foot, a bend.

ankyle- bent, crooked

Annulus (AN-yoo-lus) the outer fibrous ring of the intervertebral disc.

annulus: diminutive of Lt. anus = ring, hence little ring.(AS anulus).

anomalo- uneven, irregular

ansa (AN-su) Lt. ansa = loop/looplike, hence ansa cervicalis loop of nerves in the neck supplying thyro-hyoid muscles.

ansa nephroni = Loop of Henle

antagonist: Gk. anti = against, and agonistes = rival, hence a muscle which may oppose an agonist. adj.- agonist.

ante- before

anteflexion: Lt. ante = before, and flexere = to bend, anterior angulation between the body and cervix of the uterus.

anterior: comparative of Lt. ante = before, in front.

Anterior (ahn-TER-ee-or) toward the belly or front of the body (in humans, see also ventral) ≠ posterior.

Anterior horn a region of the SC grey matter containing the cell bodies of motor neuron. (see also the ventral horn).

Anterior root the structure emerging from the SC on its anterior aspect that contains axons of motor neurons (see also the ventral root).

Anterior pituitary gland the portion of the pituitary gland at the base of the brain composed of glandular epithelium (see also adenohypophysis).

antero- anterior, forward

anteversion: Lt. ante = before, and versum = turned, hence, the anterior angulation b/n cervix uteri & the vagina.

anti- against, combating

Antibiotic (ant-EE-BYE-o-tic) a substance which can be ingested and used to kill micro-organisms, specifically bacteria in the body.

anthrax: Gk. coal, carbuncle – infectious bacterial disease transmitted to man via contact with infected animals.

Antibody / Antigen, proteins involved in the immune system – antibodies Abs are produced by the body in reaction to antigens Ags proteins or materials found on the surface of foreign bodies introduced to the body forming the antibody-antigen complex.

antrum: Gk. antron - cave, hence a space in a bone or organ.

anulus: diminutive of Lt. anus = ring, hence little ring. (AS annulus)

Anuric- (an-YOU-ric) absence of urine production

Anus (AY-nus) the distal end and outlet of the rectum.

anus: Lt. = ring, adj.- anal.

Aorta (AY-OR-tah) the main trunk of the systemic circulatory circuit. It originates from the L ventricle.

Aortic semilunar valve - one of 4 heart valves, it consists of 3 cusps that are attached to the wall of the aorta near its origin from the L ventricle.= aortic valve.

ap- toward , near to

ap- away from, derived from, separation

Aperture (a-PET-tyuu-a) an opening or space b/n bones or w/n a bone.

Apex (A-pehks)- the extremity of a conical or pyramidal structure. The apex of the heart is the rounded, inferior most tip that points to the L side.

apocrine: Gk apo = from –crine = secrete specific type of exocrine sweat gland, which sloughs off the top of the cells

aponeurosis: Gk. apo = from, & neuron = tendon (later applied to nerve cell & its fibres), used for sheet-like tendons. Adj.- aponeurotic

apophysis: Gk. apo = from, and physis = growth, a bony process - the articular process of a vertebra; adj.- apophysial.

Apoptosis (ap-oh-TOE-sis) individual cell death.

apoptosis: Gk. apo = from, ptosis = fall to describe the phenomenon of individual cell death in an organ.

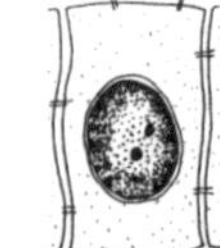
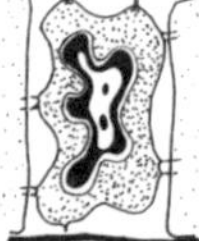
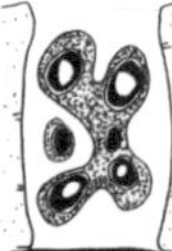

appendage: Lt. appendere = to hang on, supplement.
appendix: Lt. appendere = to hang on, supplement.
apposition: Lt. appositus = placed at, hence, in contact, in juxtaposition.
aqueduct: Lt. aqua = water, and ductus = drawn or led off, a channel for conducting fluid, e.g. the cerebral aqueduct of the midbrain, which transmits fluid from the 3rd to the 4th ventricle.

Aqueous (AY-kwee-us) water, transparent fluid.

Arachnoid (a-RAK-noyd) the middle of 3 CT coverings (meninges) of the brain & the SC. (Pia, Arachnoid & Dura from inner to outer layers).
arachnoid: adj.Gk. arachne = spider, and eidos = shape or form, hence like a spider's web. This middle layer of the three meninges is spread web-like over the brain.

Arbor branching treelike

Areata (ARY-ar-tah) patchy

arch- chief, first, beginning,
arcuate: Lt. arcuatum = curved or arched.
arcus: Lt. an arch, Lt. arcuatum = curved or arched area: a part of a surface, also used to describe the opaque ring around the iris seen in various diseases.
areata/areatus: Lt. circumscribed areas, cf alopecia areata - specific areas eg. of baldness.
areola: Lt. small, open space.

Areolar (a-REE-oh-lar) a type of CT with sparse protein fibres in the matrix (loose CT).
argyria (arj-I-ree-ah) Lt: argyr- Lt. silver.
argyrophillic (arj-I-roh-fil-ik) Lt. argyr- silver + phallic- loving = tissue or cells which have an affinity with silver salts and stain black such as Nerve tissue.
arm: the upper limb, between shoulder and elbow.

Arrector pili (ah-REK-tor PI-lee) muscle fibres attached to hair w/n the skin.
arrector: Lt. adrectus = raised, hence, arrector pili = a hair raising muscle.
artefact AS artifact.

Arteriole (ar-TEER-ee-ol) a small tributary from a larger artery that delivers blood to a capillary.

Arteriosclerosis (ar-TEER-ee-oh-scler-OH-sis) disease of the arteries where the walls harden ± calcification

Artery (AR-ter-ee) a BV that carries blood away from the heart.
artery: Lt. arteria (to take away)

A B C D E F G H I J K L M N O P Q R S T U V W X Y Z

Arthritis (AR-th-rite-tis) Lt. arthus = joint, - itis = inflammation - inflammation of joints.

arthrodesis: Lt. arthro = joint, desis = to stiffen, hence the fusion of a joint or the stiffening of a joint.

Articular cartilage (ar-TIH-kyoo-lar KAR-ti-lej) the cartilage that covers the end of a bone, where it forms a joint with another bone.

Articulation (ar-tik'-yoo-LAY-shun) = joint, which is a point of contact b/n 2 opposing bones.

articulation: Lt. artus = joint, hence, articulate - to form a joint.

Artifact (AH-te-fact) AS **Artefact**

artifact: Lt art = art, factum = made – any distortion or introduction of an object in Histology, Radiology processing of specimens - not natural.

arytenoid: Gk. arytaina = pitcher, and eidos = shape or form, the arytenoid cartilage curves like a spout.

as- toward, near to

Ascending colon (ah-SEN-ding KO-lun) a segment of the large intestine that extends from the caecum to the transverse colon = Right colon.

Ascites (ASS-cite-ees) accumulation of fluid in the peritoneal cavity.

aspect: a view of more than one surface.

aspera: Lt. rough.

Asphyxia (ASS-fix-ee-ya) suffocation, anoxia with an increase in CO^2

asterion: Gk. asterios = starry.

asthen- weak, weakness

Astrocyte (AS-tro-site) a neuroglial cell type common in the CNS, particularly the brain. Astrocytes are believed to form a structural framework b/n neurons, BV, and other neuroglial cells by their attachments. They are also capable of impulse transmission.

astrocyte: Gk. astron = star, and kytos = cell, hence a star-shaped (neuroglial) cell.

ataxia: Gk. a = negative, and taxis = order, hence inability to co-ordinate the voluntary muscles.

Atelectasis (AT-e-lec-TAY-sis) incomplete opening of the lungs

atelectasis : GK. ateles = incomplete, ektasis = opening – incomplete opening used in the pulmonary system to indicate under inflated lungs.

atlas: Gk. atlao = I sustain. Atlas was the mythical god who sustained the globe on his shoulders. The 1st vertebra sustains the skull, and its upper surface bears 2 concavities.

Atheroma (ath-e–ROH-mah) = Atherosis lipid deposits in the intima of the arteries, part of the process of atherosclerosis.

atheroma: Gk athere = gruel/porridge, oma = tumor – gruel-like lumps on the inner surface of the arteries.
atopy: Gk = atopis out of place
atresia: Gk. a = negative, and tresis = a hole, an absence or closure of a body orifice or tubular organ

atreto- closed, imperforate

Atrium (A-tree-um) One of 2 superior chambers of the heart. pl. - atria. (A-tree-Uh)
atrium: Lt. = entrance hall, adj.- atrial.

Atrophy (a-TROH-fee) wasting away deterioration of a tissue or organ from lack of use or food.

Atypical (AY-tip-i-cal) not usual - often used to describe possible cancerous cells or tissue.
auditory: Lt. audire = to hear, hence, pertaining to the ear.
auricle: Lt. auricula = a little ear - part of the external ear.
auricular - ear-shaped.
auscultate: Lt. ausculto = to listen to.

auto- self, spontaneous

Autolysis (OR-tol-e-sis): auto Gk. auto = self, lysis = dissolving - hence the process of self destruction of a cell or tissue.

Autopsy (OR-top-see) the examination ± dissection of a body after death - usually to investigate cause of death / verify the diagnosis.
autonomic: adj.Gk. auto = self, & nomos = law, hence self-regulating.

aux- help, growth, increase

Axial (AKS-ee-el) refers to the head and trunk (vertebrae, ribs and sternum) of the body - axial skeleton including the skull and the vertebral column.
axilla: Lt. armpit.
axis: Lt. axis = the central line of a body or part thereof, especially the imaginary line around which rotation takes place adj. axial.

Axon (AKS-on) a long process of a neuron that carries a nerve impulse away from the cell body.
axon: Lt. axis = axis, hence the main process of a neuron conducting impulses away from the cell body.
azygos: adj. Gk. a = negative, and zygos = paired, hence, unpaired.

B

balan GK = penis

bar- pressure

barbae Gk = beard

bary- low, heavy, deep, difficult

Basement membrane (BM) a thin layer of extracellular material and CT stroma that underlies epithelium.

basi- foundation, base

basilar: adj. Lt. basis = base.

basilic: adj. Gk. basilikos = royal (king-sized).

Basophil (BAS-oh-fil) a type of WBC that is characterized by large cytoplasmic granules that stain blue with basic dyes.

Benign (BEE-nine), (Fr benignus = kind) not harmful or dangerous, ≠ malignant, indicating a mild disease or a mild non-malignant cancer.

Beta (BEE- tah) **cell** a cell in the pancreatic islets of Langerhans that secretes the H, insulin.

bi- twice, two, double (see di)

biceps: Lt. bis = double, and caput = head, hence 2-headed, adj.- bicipital.

bifid: adj.Lt. bis = double, & findo = to split.

bifurcate: Lt. bis = double, & furco = fork, hence to divide into two.

bilateral: Lt. bi = two, lateral = side, hence, pertaining to two (both) sides.

bin- twice, two, double

bio- life

Biopsy (BYE-op-see) removal of a piece of living tissue for examination.

bipennate: adj, Lt. bis = double, and pinna = feather, hence converging from 2 sides.

blast- undifferentiated, immature

blepharo- eyelid

Blind spot a region of the retina where no photoreceptive cells are present, due to the exit point of the Optic N.

Body cavity a space in the body that is internally lined by a membrane, & contains structures including organs.

Bone a CT that contains a hardened matrix of mineral salts and collagen fibres. Its cells include osteocytes, which are embedded within lacunae, and the free-roaming osteoblasts and osteoclasts.

border: see margin.

Bowman's capsule (BO-manz CAP-sewl) the part of the kidney nephron that surrounds the glomerulus, (see glomerular capsule).

Brachial (BRAY-kee-al) arm, mainly to do with the upper arm

brachiocephalic: Lt. brachium = arm, and Gk. kephale = head, a BV related to the upper limb and head.

brachium: Lt. = arm, adj.- brachial.

brachy- short

brady- slow ≠ tachy

Brain stem the inferior portion of the brain that consists of the midbrain, pons, and medulla oblongata.

branchia: Gk. = gills, adj.- branchial.

bregma: Gk. = moist, referring to the site of the anterior fontanelle (ie a little fountain) the site of junction of the coronal & sagittal sutures, where the brain can be felt pulsating in infancy.

brevi- short

brevis: Lt. = short - cf. brief.

bronch- windpipe

Bronchiectasis (BRONG-kee-ek-tas-is) chronic dilatation or opening of the bronchi in the lung.

Bronchiole (BRONG-kee-ol) a small bronchus - a series of small tubes that arise as branches from tertiary bronchi w/n each lung (bronchi have cartilage in their walls, bronchioles do not).

Bronchitis (brong-KITE-is) inflammation of the bronchi

Bronchus (BRONG-kus) any one of the air passageways that carry air between the trachea and the bronchioles. pl.- bronchi. adj. bronchial.

Brunner's glands mucous glands located w/n the submucosa of the small intestine.

buccal: adj.Lt. bucca = cheek.

buccinator: Lt. = trumpeter - this is the muscle which blows air out from the cheek

bulb: Lt. = bulbus, bolbus, rounded object

Bulimia (BULL-ee-mee-ya) Lt. bous = ox + limos = hunger–hence huge episodic bingeing of food eating followed by self = induced vomiting or excessive exercising.

bulbus: Lt. = bulb or onion.

bulla: Lt. = bubble.

bunion: Lt. = bounion = turnip

Bursa (BER-suh): Gk. = a purse, hence a flattened sac containing a film of fluid. pl bursae.

C

cac- (KAK) bad, diseased, deformed , ill

Caecum (SEE-kuhm) the proximal end of the large intestine which receives the terminal ileum of the small intestine. AS Cecum.

caecum: Lt. = blind. (AS cecum)

caen- (SEEN) new recent

calcaneus: Lt. calx = heel, hence the bone of the heel.

calcar: Lt. = a spur.

calcar avis: Lt. the spur of a bird, hence a spur-like elevation.

calcarine: Lt. calcar = spur, hence spur-shaped.

Calculus (KAL-kew-lus) generally referring to stones in the renal system – bladder

calculus: Lt. calculus = pebble, small stone, hence a concretion occurring w/in the organism made up at least in part of mineral salts (pl. - calculi).

calf: the soft tissue swelling at the back of the leg.

calyx (KAY-lix): Lt. = a wine-cup (plural – calices (KAY-li-sees) alternative spelling calyx.

calix: Lt. = a wine-cup (plural - calices) alternative spelling calyx.

callosum: Lt. callum = hard.

calotte: calvaria from which the base has been removed

callous Gk. = hard (AS callus).

Callus a disorganized pattern of woven bone formed after a fracture.

calotte: calvaria from which the base has been removed.

Calvaria (KAL-vair-ree-uh) refers to the cranium w/o the facial bones attached

calvaria: Lt. calva = bald head, part of the skull containing the brain- i.e. cranium minus the facial skeleton.

calyx: Lt. = a wine-cup (plural - calyces) found in the renal pelvis

canal: Lt. canalis = a water-pipe or canal.

Canaliculus (kan-al-LIK-yew-lus) a small channel w/n compact bone tissue that connects lacunae. pl. canaliculi. diminutive of canal.

cancellous: adj.Lt. cancelli = grating or lattice.

Cancer (KAN –ser) group of diseases where cells grow out of control

canine: adj.Lt. canis = dog.

canthus: Gk. kanthos = angle b/n ends of rims.

Capillary (kar-PIL-lar'-ee) a microscopic BV = that interconnects arterioles with venules. The capillary wall is a single cell layer in thickness, and is the only site of nutrient diffusion b/n the BS & body cells.

capillary: Lt. capillaris = hair-like, a very thin BV.

capitate: adj.having a caput from Lt. capitis = of a head (q.v.).

capitulum: diminutive of caput, Lt. = head.

Capsule (KAP-syoo-l) an enclosing membrane.

capsule: Lt. capsa = box, hence an enclosing sheet.

caput: Lt. = head. Capitis - of a head, adj.- capitate = having a head (c.f. decapitate).

caput medusae: Lt. caput = head, Medusa = Gk. mythical female with ugly snake like hair.

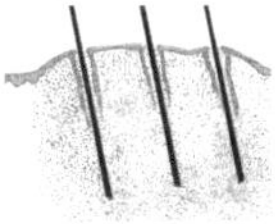

Carbuncle (KAR-bunk-el) compound necrotizing inflammation of the skin ± subcutaneous tissues - (multiheaded pimple).

Cancer (KAN-ser): (Lt. crab - describing originally the crab-like invasion of cancer cells spreading out into normal tissue) – malignant neoplasms.

Carcinogen (KAR-sin-oh-jen) material which leads to cancer formation.

Carcinoid description of a tumor or agentaffin cells in the GIT or lungs, slow growing and covered in mucosa.

Carcinoma (KAR-sin-oh-mah) a malignant growth originating from epithelial cells.

Carcinoma - *in situ* preinvasive cancer still lying in the confines of normal tissue not having broken through the BM but with neoplastic changes.

Cardiac muscle (KAR-dee-ahk MUS-ehl) one of 3 types of muscle tissue. It is characterized by striations and involuntary contractions, and makes up the bulk of the heart wall.

cardinal: Lt. cardinalis = principal, of primary importance.

Carina (KAR-rin-ah) the point of bifurcation of the 2 primary bronchi in the lung.

carina: Lt. = a keel.

carneae: Lt. carnea = fleshy. (kar-nee)

carotid: Gk. karoo, = to put to sleep; compression of the common or internal carotid artery causes coma.

carpus (KAR-pus): Gk. = wrist, adj.- carpal.

Cartilage (KAWR-tih-lehj) a type of CT characterized by the presence of a matrix containing a dense distribution of proteins & a thickened ground substance. The matrix is mainly secreted by chondroblasts.

cartilage: Lt. = gristle; adj.- cartilaginous.

caruncle: diminutive of Lt. caro = flesh, hence, a small fleshy elevation.

caseation (KAY-see-ay-shon): Lt. cheese, hence a form of necrosis or tissue death resulting in a cheeselike formation.

Cataract (kat-a-RAkT) : Gk. katarraktes = waterfall, a thickening on the lens of the eye which affects vision either partially or completely often making it look blurry.

cauda: Lt. = tail, adj.- caudate - having a tail.

cauda equina: Lt. = a horse's tail.

caudal: Lt. cauda = tail, hence toward the tail, inferior (in human anatomy). Note legs are inferior not caudal.

caudate: Lt. cauda = tail, hence having a tail.

cava: Lt. cavum = cave, hollow.

cavernous: Lt. containing caverns or cave-like spaces.

Cavity: (KAV-it-ee) an open area or sinus within a bone or formed by 2 or more bones. (in dentistry a pathological hollow in the bone - tooth).

cavity: Lt. cavitas = a hollow.

cavum: Lt. = cave.

cecum: Lt. = blind. (AS caecum)

celiac: adj.Gk. koilia = belly. (AS coeliac)

Cell (SELL) the basic living unit of multicellular organisms.

Cell body the portion of a neuron containing the nucleus and much of the cytoplasm. (also = the soma).

celom: (SEE-lohm): Gk. koilos = a hollow (AS coelom)

cen- general, common - new, recent (sen)

centi- hundredth part, hundred (sen-tee)

Central fovea (FO-vee-ah) a small depression in the centre of the macula lutea of the retina. It contains cone cells (only), and is the area of optimal visual acuity (clearest vision).

Central nervous system (**CNS**) A major division of the nervous system (NS) that contains the brain & spinal cord (SC).

Central vein when pertaining to the liver, the central vein is a vein located in the center of a liver lobule that conveys blood from the hepatocytes to the hepatic vein.

Centriole (SEHN-tree-ol) cylindrical structures within the cytoplasm of a cell, consisting of microtubules, which play a role in cell division.

central: adj.Lt. centrum = centre.

centrum: Lt. = centre.

cephal- head

Cephalic (KEF–al-ik) pertaining to the head.

cephalic: adj.Gk. kephale = head.

cer- wax (ser)

cerat- cornea / horny tissue (kerat)

Cerebellum (ser'-eh-BELL-uhm) a functional region of the hindbrain located inferior to the cerebrum. It co-ordinates muscle movement.

cerebellum: diminutive of Lt. cerebrum = brain.

Cerebral cortex the outer layer of the cerebrum, which is composed of grey matter.

Cerebrum (SER-ee-bruhm) the largest functional region of the brain, it is the convoluted mass that lies superior to all other parts of the brain. It is the main site of integration of sensory & motor impulses.

cerebrum: Lt. = brain, adj.- cerebral.

Ceroid (SE-royd) waxlike substance found in pathological tissues – e.g. cirrhotic livers.

cerumen: Lt. cera = wax.

cervical: adj.Lt. cervix = neck, pertaining to the neck.

Cervix (SER-viks) the narrow, constricted, fibrous part of the uterus that is b/n the vagina & the body of the uterus.

cervix: Lt. = neck, adj.- cervical.

Chalazion (kal-AYZ-ee-on) : Lt. Gk. chalaze = small lump, small tumor of the eyelid due to build up of the mucous glands = tarsal cyst = meibomian cyst.

chancr- canerous, abnormal growth, rotting (kankr-)

cheil- lip (cheel-)

chiasma: Gk. kiasma = cross. (The Gk. letter chi = c) eg optic chiasma. (KEYE-az-muh)

chemo- relating to chemistry, chemically induced (keem-oh)

Chemotaxis (KEEM-oh-tax-is) – cellular phenomenon of moving towards or away from specific areas due to the chemical present.

chiro- hand (kyro-)

chol- gall, bile (kohl)

cholang- bile vessel or passage (kohl-ange)

chondra- cartilage (kondra-)

chondral: adj.Gk. chondros = cartilage.

Chondrium (KON-dree- um) the cartilage adj. chondria, chondral

Chondrocyte (KON-droh-site) a mature cartilage cell.

Chondroitin sulfate (kon-DROI-tin SUL-fate) a semisolid material forming part of the EC matrix in certain CT.

chorda: Lt. = cord.

chori- protective membrane (kor-ee-)

Chorea (KOR-ee-uh) (Gk. choriea - a dance) convulsive involuntary

A B **C** D E F G H I J K L M N O P Q R S T U V W X Y Z

irregular nervous movements

Choroid (KO-royd) part of the vascular tunic covering of the eyeball. It lines most of the internal surface of the sclera, forming the middle layer of the wall of the eye.

Chorion ((KAW-ree-on): Gk. chorios = membrane – membranes around the foetus.

Choroid plexus (KO-royd PLEKS-sus) a mass of specialized capillaries in the ventricles of the brain, from which CSF is produced.

choroid: adj.Gk. chorion = skin and eidos = shape or form, hence, like a membrane.

chrom- coloured (krohm-)

Chromatin (KROH-mah-tin) the mass of genetic material in the nucleus of a cell, consisting mostly of DNA. It is only visible during interphase.

Chromosome (KRO-mo-som) one of the structures (46 in human cells) within the cell nucleus that contains genetic material. Chromosomes become visible during cell division.

chron- time (kron-)

Chronic (Kron-ik) long standing ≠ acute, generally used in disease states.

chyle- digested fats (ky-lee)

chyle: Gk. = juice. also chyli: Gk. = juice.

cili- eyelash (sil-ee)

cilia- hair (sil-ee-ah)

ciliary: adj.Lt. cilia = eyelashes.

Cilia (SIL-ee-ah) a hairlike process associated with a cell that is a modification of the plasma membrane. Its movement generates a flow of fluid (usually mucus) in the extracellular environment. sing. = cilium.

cilium: Lt. = eyelid, hence, an eyelash; adj.- ciliary, or ciliated. pl. - cilia.

cine- movement (sin-ee)

cingulum: Lt. girdle or belt, adj.- cingulate.

circum- around , surrounding (SER-kum)

circumflex: Lt. circum = around, and flexere = to bend, hence, bend or bent around.

cirrho- yellow, orange (si-roh)

Cirrhosis: Gk. yellow - but also refers to the hardening of the liver, always pathological.

cis- on this side (sis)

cisterna: Lt. = a cistern.

claustrum: Lt. clausum = closed, hence a barrier.

clavicle: diminutive of Lt. clavis = key - old Roman keys were S-shaped.

cleid- clavicle (klyde-)

cleido: Gk., cleis = key, a combining form denoting relationship to the clavicle.

cleist- closed (klyst-)

clinoid: adj.Gk. kline = bed, eidos = shape or form, hence, like a bed-post.

clist- closed

clivus: Lt. = slope (c.f. declivity).

Clone: Gk. slip – referring to probation by cutting a slip from a plant, hence reproduction and propogation via a single cell.

co- with, together (koh)

Coagulation (KOH-ag-you-lay-shon) (Lt. coaulo - to curdle as in milk curdling) process of clotting turning from a liquid to a solid or semi-solid.

coccyx: Gk. kokkyx = cuckoo, whose bill the coccyx resembles.

Cochlea (KOK-lee-ah) the portion of the inner ear which contains the receptors of hearing – the organ of Corti.

cochlea: Lt. = snail, hence the spiral cochlea, adj.- cochlear.

coeliac: adj.Gk. koilia = belly. (AS celiac).

coen- general, common

col- with, together

coli: Lt. = of the colon.

Collagen (KOL-a-jen) a protein that is an abundant component of CT.

collateral: adj.Lt. con = together, & latus = side, hence, alongside.

colli: genetive (possessive case) of collum, Lt. = neck

colliculus: diminutive of Lt. collis = hill.

collum: Lt. = neck (cf. collar).

Colon (KOH-lun) the large intestine, containing the ascending, transverse, descending & sigmoid sections.

colon: Gk. kolon = large intestine.

colp- vaginal (kohlp)

columna: Lt. = column, or pillar.

com- together, with

Coma (KOH-mah) (Gk koma = sleep) - depressed state of consciousness & ability to respond to stimuli.

Comedo/comedone- (KOM-e-doh) non-inflammatory lesion of the skin – blackhead / whitehead

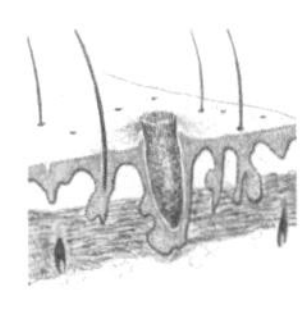

A B C D E F G H I J K L M N O P Q R S T U V W X Y Z

A B **C** D E F G H I J K L M N O P Q R S T U V W X Y Z

comitans: adj.Lt. = accompanying.
commissure: Lt. con = together, & missum = sent, fibres which cross b/n symmetrical parts.
communicans: adj.Lt. = communicating.

Compact bone one of 2 types of bone tissue, it is characterized by a dense EC matrix filled with mineral salts & collagen arranged in lamellae that surround a central osteonic (Haversian) canal (= dense bone).

con- together, with (Kon)

concha: Lt. = shell. pl. conchae – pertaining to shell shapes as in the ear and nose.

Condyle (KON-dile) a rounded enlargement or process possessing an articular surface.

condyle: Gk. kondylos = knuckle.

Cone cell a photoreceptor in the retina of the eye that is involved in colour vision and high visual acuity.

congenital (KON-jen-it-al) present from birth
conjunctiva: Lt. con = with, and junctus = joined (cf. junction).

Connective tissue (kon-EK-tiv Tishh-ew) (CT) one of the 4 basic types of tissue in the body. It is characterized by an abundance of EC material with relatively few cells, and functions in the support and binding of body structures.

conoid: Gk. konoeides = resembling a cone, cone shape
constrictor: Lt. con = together, and strictum = drawn tight, hence, producing narrowing.
contour: Gk. tornos = lathe, hence a line which turns - an outline.

contra- opposite against

contralateral: Lt. contra = against, latus = side, the opposite side (≠ ipsilateral).
conus: Lt. = cone, conus medullaris - the lower end of the spinal cord

cor-heart

coracoid: adj. = like a crow's beak.

Cornea (KOR-nee-ah) the transparent, anterior portion of the fibrous tunic covering the eye, derived from 2 germinal layers.

cornea: Lt. cornu = horn, hence, the dense transparent tissue forming the front of the eyeball.
corniculate: Lt. = shaped like a small horn.
cornu: Lt. = horn.
corona: Lt. = crown. adj.- coronary or coronal; hence a coronal plane is parallel to the main arch of a crown which passes from ear to ear (c.f. coronal suture).

Corona radiata (koh-RO-nah ra-dee-AR-tah) several layers of follicle cells that form a protective mantle around the secondary oocyte.

Coronal (kor-RO-nal) **plane** a plane that extends vertically to divide the body into anterior & posterior portions. Also = the frontal plane.

coronary: adj. Lt. = crown, hence, encircling like a crown.

coronoid: adj. shaped like a crown.

corp- body (korp)

corpus: Lt. = body, pl.- corpora – pertaining to the body or the main part of the organ.

Corpus luteum (KOR-puhs LOO-tee-uhm) a structure w/n the ovary that forms from a ruptured Graafian follicle and functions as an endocrine gland by secreting female hormones.

Corpuscle (KOR-puhs-ehl) used to describe a small body contained w/n a sac, as in red corpuscle (RBC) small package of haemoglobin (see also renal corpuscle).

corpuscle: Lt. = a little body.

corrugator: Lt. con = together, and ruga = wrinkle, hence a muscle that produces wrinkles.

Cortex (KOR-tehks) the outer portion of an organ. (≠ medulla)

cortex: Lt. = bark, adj.– cortical.

cost- rib (kost)

costa: Lt. = rib. adj.– costal.

coxa: Lt. = hip, hence os coxae = the hip bone.

Cranium (KRAYN-ee-um) consists of all the bones of the skull with the exception of the mandible.

cranium: Gk. kranion = skull. adj. cranium.

cremaster: Gk. = suspender, hence the muscle which suspends the testis.

Crenation (kre-NAY-shun) the shrinkage of a cell caused by contact with an hypotonic solution.

Crescent (KR-es-ent) crown of epithelial cells – as seen in glomerulonephritis on Bowman's capsule.

Crest (KR-est) a narrow ridge.

cribriform: adj.Lt. cribrum = sieve, hence, sieve-like.

cricoid: adj.– ring-like, circular.

crista: Lt. = crest, crista galli = the (median) crest of a cock.

Cristae sensory organs of dynamic equilibrium, which are located w/n the ampullae of the inner ear.

Crown the part of a tooth that is exposed, and covered with enamel.

cruciate: adj.Lt. crux = cross, hence, crossed like the letter X.

crur- leg (kroo-r)
crus: Lt. = leg, plural - crura.
cryo- cold freezing
crypt- hidden, covered occult
cubital: adj.Lt. cubitus = elbow.
cuboid: adj.Gk. kuboides = cube-shaped.
culmen: Lt. = summit (c.f. culminate).
cuneate: adj.Lt. = a wedge.
cuneiform: adj.Lt. cuneus = wedge, hence wedge-shaped. *See also sphen.*
cuneus: Lt. = a wedge, adj.– cuneate.

Cupula a gelatinous mass located w/n the ampullae of the inner ear. It shifts in response to changes in the position of the head. This shift generates an impulse, which is interpreted in the brain as dynamic equilibrium.
cupola: Lt. = little dome. / cupula: Lt. = little dome. (AS cupula)
cusp: Lt. cuspis = a pointed elevation.

cutis- skin (kew-tis)
cutaneous: adj.Lt. cutis = skin.

Cutaneous (kew-TAY-nee-us) **membrane** one of the 3 types of epithelial membranes found in the body, it is also known as the skin.

Cyanosis (SEYE-an –oh-sis): Gk. kyanos = blue material, hence blueness of the skin, or elsewhere due to the lack of oxygen.

cymbo- boat shaped (sim-boh)
cyrt- bent, curved
cyst- sac bladder (sist-)
cyst: Gk. kystis = bladder, adj.- cystic.
cyt-/cyte- cell (site-) mature cell type

Cytokinesis (SI-to-ky-nee-sis) the division of the cytoplasm as a part of the process in mitosis resulting in 2 equal daughter cells.

Cytology (SI-tol-oh-jee) the study of individual cells.

Cytoplasm (SI-to-plazm) the material of a cell located w/n the plasma membrane & outside the nuclear membrane, containing the cellular organelles.

Cytosol (SI-toh-sol) the thickened fluid of the cytoplasm. It lies outside the cellular organelle membranes.

Cytoskeleton (si'-to-SKEHL-eh-ton) the complex supportive network of microtubules & microfilaments in the cytoplasm.

D

dactyl- digit, finger, toe (dak-til)
dartos: Gk. = flayed or skinned.
de- remove, undoing, reversal, depriving, freeing from
dec- ten, tenth (dess)
declive: Lt. declivitas = slope (cf. clivus).
decussation: Lt. decussatus = crossed like the letter X.
Deep a directional term meaning away from the surface of the body. (≠ superficial)
Deep fascia (FASH-ee-ah) a sheet of CT covering the external surface of a muscle (also = the epimysium).
deferens: adj.Lt. = carrying down.
Degeneration- retrogressive cell & tissue changes short of necrosis.
deglutition: Lt. deglutire = to swallow, hence the act of swallowing.
dehiscence: Lt. de = away, hiscere = to gape, hence, a separation, a splitting away (as in wounds).
deka- multiple of ten
deltoid: adj. Gk. delta (D), the capital letter has a triangular shape (c.f. the delta of the Nile).
dem- people, population (dem)
demi- half (dem-ee)
Dendrite (DEN-dryt) a cytoplasmic extension from the cell body of a neuron which carries a nerve impulse towards the cell body.
dendrite: or dendron, Gk. = a tree, hence like the branches of a tree
dendro- branching, treelike
dens: Lt. = tooth (c.f. dentist), adj.- dental.
Dense irregular connective tissue a CT that contains an EC matrix densely populated with collagen fibres, which extend in irregular directions - found in the dermis of skin.
Dense regular connective tissue a CT that contains a matrix densely populated with collagen fibres, which extend in parallel directions. It is the main component of tendons and ligaments.
dent- teeth
dentate: Lt. dens = tooth, hence, having a toothed margin.
denticulate: Lt. dens = tooth, hence, having small tooth-like projections.
Dentin (DEN-teen) the bonelike material forming the bulk of a tooth.
dentine: from Lt. dens = tooth; the substance of the tooth surrounding the pulp.

Deoxyribonucleic acid (dee-ohk'-see-ry-bo-nyoo-KLAY-ik AH-sihd) (**DNA**) a nucleic acid in the shape of a double helix that contains the genetic information necessary for protein synthesis.

depress: Lt. de = prefix implying descent, and pressum = pressed, hence to press down.

depression = downward movement or a concavity on a surface.

Depressor (DEE-press-ohr) muscle which pushes down (≠ levator).

dermatome: Gk. derma = skin, tome = a cutting or division, a segment of skin supplied by a single spinal ganglion.

derm(o)- skin

dermato- skin

Dermis (DER-mis) the layer of the skin lying deep to the epidermis and composed of dense irregular CT.

dermis: Gk. = skin, adj.- dermal.

Dermatitis (derm-u-TEYE-tis) any skin inflammatory process – see also Eczema

Dermatome (DERM-at-tohm) section of sensation on skin corresponce to the distribution of a N root - note there is a lot of overlap. *See P189*

Descending colon (dee-SEN-ding KO-lun) the segment of the large intestine b/n the transverse colon & the sigmoid colon (= Left colon).

Desquammation (dee-SKWAR-may-shon) the shedding of the Stratum Corneum of the skin (see also Exfoliation)

detrusor: Lt. detrusio = thrust away.

desmo- ligament

deuter- secondary, second

di- two, twice, double, reversal, separation, apart from

dia- through, across, between, apart, complete

Diabetes (DYE-uh-beet-eez) (Gk: diabetes = a siphon) - to pass through - referring to the polyuria - huge urine output - of diabetes mellitus.

Diagnosis (DYE-ag-noh-sis) (Gk: a deciding – decision) a determination of the nature of the disease.

diaphragm: Gk. dia = across, and phragma = wall, hence, a partition, adj - diaphragmatic (see phrenic).

Diaphysis (di-AH-fih-sihs) the shaft of a long bone.

diaphysis: Gk. dia = apart, and physis = growth, hence the body of a long bone b/n the growing regions near the ends.

diastole: Gk. dia = apart, & stellein = sending, hence sending the walls of the heart apart, i.e. relaxation or dilatation. adj.- diastolic.

diencephalon: Gk. dia = between, & enkephalos = brain, in general the structures surrounding the 3rd ventricle. adj.- diencephalic.

Differentiation (DIF-er-ent-she-ay-shon) the process of changing from one kind of tissue or cell to another, generally to a more complex form.

digastric: adj. Gk. dia = double, & gaster = belly, hence, 2 - bellied (as in muscles).

digit: Lt. digitus = a finger or toe, usually excepting the pollex (thumb) or hallux (big toe), adj.- digital.

diplo- double, twin

diplopia: Gk. diploos = double, & opsis = vision, hence double vision

diploë: Gk. = fold, the cancellous bone b/n the inner and outer tables of the skull, adj.- diploic.

dis- apart from, two, twice, double , reversal, separation, difficult, wrong

discus: Lt. = disc. adj. discoid

Disease: – Eng. dis- ease, lack of comfort , anything limiting health and comfort of the organism

Dissection (DYE-sek-shon) to cut up to carve in a systematic way

dissection: Lt. disssecare = to cut up, from dis = apart, sectum = cut (c.f. anatomy).

Distal (DIS-tahl) away from the middle of the body or the axis or core of the body proximal

distal: adj. Lt. di = apart, and stans = standing, hence, standing apart, implying farther from a given point.

Distal convoluted tubule a segment of the renal tubule (of the kidney nephron) that extends from the loop of Henle to the collecting duct. Its pathway is very twisted.

diverticulum: Lt. = by-road, hence a blind tubular process or sac

dolor : Lt. = pain

Dorsal (DOR-sal) a directional term indicating toward the back side, or posterior.

dorsal: adj.Lt. dorsum = back.

Dorsal root the sensory branch of a spinal nerve which connects with the SC.

dorsum: Lt. = back.

ductus: Lt. = duct.

Ductus deferens (DUK-tuhs DEF-er-ehnz) the tube that conducts sperm from the epididymis in the testes to the ejaculatory duct. (also = vas deferens, and seminal duct).

duo- two

Duodenum (dew-OH-den-uhm) the first segment of the small intestine extending from the pyloric valve to the jejunum.

duodenum: Lt. duodenarius = twelve, because it is 12 fingerbreadths long.

dura: adj.Lt. = hard (cf. durable); dura mater, the tough covering membrane of the CNS.

dy- two

dynam- power energy (dye-nam)

Dynamic equilibrium the sensation of rapid movements, mostly of the head.

dysphagia: Gk. dys = difficult, and phagein = to eat, hence, difficulty in swallowing.

dys- difficult, painful, abnormal

Dysentry (DIS-en-tree) (Gk. dys- = bad - enteros = bowels) referring to inflammation of the bowel and resulting in blood and mucous in the frequent bowel movements - serious possibility of dehydration from fluid loss in this area.

dysphagia: Gk. dys = difficult, & phagein = to eat, hence, difficulty in swallowing.

Dystrophy (DIS-troh-fee) irregular abnormal growth.

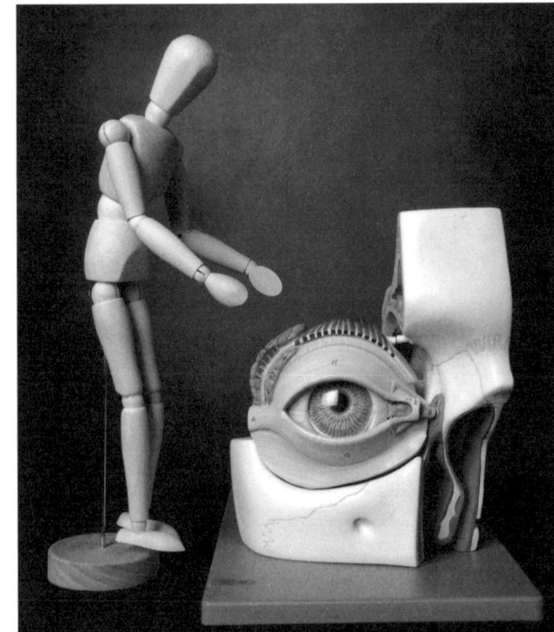

E

A B C D E F G H I J K L M N O P Q R S T U V W X Y Z

e- outside, external, out, protrude, over, away, less

ec- outside, out, to protrude over, away, less / house

Eccrine (EHK-krin) the common type of sweat gland found all over the body that functions in the maintenance of body temperature.

Eclampsia (EE-klam-see-uh) Gk. eklampsis = shining forth - convulsions not due to epilepsy or other neural conditions - generally referring to fits in the last trimester of pregnancy due to renal ± hepatic conditions.

Ecthyma (ek-THIGH-muh)-Gk. ekthyma ulcerative pyoderma infection - (gen streptococcal infection) at the site of minor trauma, mainly shins, dorsum of the feet - causing scar formation.

ecto- outer, out of place

echin- spine or thornlike processes (ee-kine)

Ectoderm (EHK-toh-derm) one of 3 primary germ layers in the developing embryo. It gives rise to the NS & to the epidermis and its derivatives.

ectoderm: Gk. ektos = outside, and derm = skin, hence, the outermost germ layer of the embryo.

- ectomy to cut out, excise surgically

ectopic: Gk. ek = out, and topos = place, hence out of place.

Eczema (EX-muh) GK ekzein = bubbling out any vesicular dermatitis

Edema (eh-DEE-mah) AS Oedema- pathological build up of fluid in tissues.

edge: border or margin of a surface.

ef- outside, out, to protrude over, away, less

efferent: adj.Lt. ex = out, & ferens = carrying, hence, conducting from.

Efferent arteriole (EHF-er-ehnt ar-TEER-ee-ole) an arteriole that transports blood away from the glomerulus of a nephron (in the kidney).

Efferent ductules (DUK-tew-lz) small coiled tubes that transport sperm from the rete testis to the epididymis.

Effluvian (EH-floo-vee-an) shedding of hair.

ejaculatory: Lt. ex = out, & jacere = to throw, hence throwing out

Elastic cartilage a type of cartilage (CT) that contains large numbers of elastic fibres in a more opaque matrix - present in the external ear, & parts of the larynx.

Elasticity (ee-lahs-TIH-sih-tee) the physiological property of tissue to return to its original shape after extension or contraction.

elbow: the junction between arm and forearm.

elevate: Lt. elevatus = raised up, hence, to raise up, and elevation = a raised part ≠ depress.

em- within, inside, into, in, on

A B C D **E** F G H I J K L M N O P Q R S T U V W X Y Z

emboliformis: adj.Gk. embolus = wedge or blocking matter.

Embolus (EM-bowl-us) Gk embolos = plug, hence a mass which travels in the BS and suddenly blocks an artery ie plugs it up, frequently resulting from a dislodged thrombus.

Embryo (EHM-bree-oh) in the human - the developing organism during the first 8 weeks of life after fertilization.

embryo: Gk. en = within, and bryein = to swell or grow, the early stage of intrauterine development.

emet- vomiting

-emia AS - aemia pertaining to blood, generally RBCs

eminence: Lt. eminens = projecting, hence, a projection (usually smooth).

emissary: adj.Lt. e = out, & emissum = sent out; emissary vein, one connecting intra- with extra-cranial venous channels.

Emphysema (em-fi- ZEEM-u) OFr. en = in, physa = bellows, an overfilling of an organ with gas - generally referring to the lung where the overfilling results in gas trapping & the destruction of alveolar tissue and subsequent lack of surface for gas exchange.

Empyema (em-PIE-ee-ma) OFr = pyon = pus, pus in a body cavity - generally in the thorax.

en- within, inside, in, on

Enamel (ee-NAM-ehl) the hardened outer covering on the crown of a tooth.

encephalon: Gk. en = within, & kephalos = head, hence, the brain.

endo- within, inside, into, on

endocardium: Gk. endo = within, and kardia = heart, the endothelial lining of the chambers of the heart.

endocranium: Gk. endo = within, and kranion = skull, the outer endostial layer of the dura mater.

Endocardium (ehn-doh-CARD-ih-um) the innermost layer of cells in the heart chambers (see endothelium).

Endochondral ossification (ehn-do-KOHN-dral OS'-if-iKA-shun) where bone tissue develops by replacing hyaline cartilage.

endocranium: Gk. = within, the skull adj. endocranial

endocrine: Gk. endo = within, : krinein = to separate, organs that ductlessly secrete products into the BS.

Endocrine gland (EHN-do-krihn gland) one of two main categories of glands, here the cellular products are secreted into the extracellular space & transported by the BS (also = ductless glands).

Endocytosis (ehn'-do-sih-TO-sihs) the active process of bulk transport of material into a cell. It includes phagocytosis and pinocytosis.

Endoderm (EN-do-derm) one of the 3 primary germ layers in an embryo, it begins as the inner layer, later forms the organs of the alimentary canal (GIT) & the respiratory tract.

endoderm: Gk. endo = within, and derm = skin, hence, the germ layer of the embryo that gives rise to the organs of the GIT, respiratory system and the lining of the BVs.

endolymph: Gk. endo = within, and Lt. lympha = clear water, hence the fluid within the membranous labyrinth of the internal ear.

Endometrium (EN-do MEE-tree-uhm) the innermost layer of the uterine wall. The endometrium undergoes changes in response to female hormones, resulting in a 28-day cycle involving menstruation during which much of the endometrium is sloughed off to be rebuilt again.

endometrium: Gk. endo = within, and metra = uterus, hence the mucosal lining of the uterine cavity.

Endomysium (ehn'-do-MY-see-uhm) the deepest layer of CT associated with muscle. It surrounds individual muscle fibres.

Endoneurium (ehn'-do-NEW-ree-uhm) the deepest layer of CT associated with a nerve. It surrounds individual nerve fibres (myelinated axons of neurons).

Endoplasmic reticulum (ehn'-do-PLAZ-mik reh-TIHK-yew-lum) (ER) a cytoplasmic organelle that consists of a series of tubules with a hollow center. It functions in the transport of cellular products (smooth ER), and as a site for protein synthesis (if ribosomes are attached, called rough ER) (see also Sarcoplasmic reticulum specially adapted for muscle fibres).

Endosteum (ehn-DOS-tee-uhm) a membrane lining the medullary cavity w/n a bone & containing osteoblasts and osteoclasts.

Endothelium (ehn'-do-THEE-lee-uhm) a layer of simple squamous epithelium lining the inside of BVs & the heart chambers (see endocardium).

endothelium: Gk. endo = within, & thele = the nipple; squamous epithelium lining the heart and BVs.

ent- within, inner

enter- to do with the gut, intestines

Eosinophil (ee'-oh-SIHN-oh-fihl) a type of granulated WBC characterized by a cytoplasm which absorbs the eosin stain.

ependyma: Gk. = an upper garment. It may refer to a vest or singlet, ie. an under-garment, hence, the lining membrane of the ventricles of the brain and central canal of the SC.

ep- upon, in addition to, beside among, on the outside, over

Ependymal (eh-PEN-di-mal) **cells** a type of neuroglial cells in the brain that line the ventricles. (also = ependymocytes).

ephilus Lt. = freckle (eh-fil-ehs)

epi-upon, in addition to, beside, among, on the outside, over

epicanthus: Gk. epi = upon, and kanthos = corner, hence, the fold of skin over the inner angle of the upper eyelid, a normal characteristic in certain races, & a congenital anomaly in others.

Epicardium (epi-KAR-dee-um) the thin outer layer of the heart wall. (also = visceral pericardium).

epicardium: Gk. epi = upon, and kardia = heart, visceral layer of serous pericardium covering the heart.

epicondyle: Gk. epi = upon, and kondylos = knuckle, a prominence on a condyle of the humerus/femur.

epicranial: adj.Gk. epi = upon, & kranion = skull, epicranial aponeurosis (galea) joining frontalis to occipitalis muscles.

Epidemic (epi-DEM-ik) Gk. demos = people, an increase in the population affected by the disease outside the normal range.

Epidermis (epi-DERM-ihs) the superficial layer of skin composed of stratified squamous epithelium.

epidermis: Gk. epi = upon, and derm = skin, hence, the most external layer of the skin.

Epididymis (epi-DID-imus) an organ in the male reproductive system that consists of a coiled tube located within the scrotum.

epididymis: Gk. epi = upon, and didymos = testis, hence, the organ perched posterosuperior to the testis.

epidural: adj.Gk. epi = upon, Lt. dura = tough, hence, external to dura mater.

epigastrium: Gk. epi = upon, & gaster = belly, hence, the upper median zone of the abdomen.

Epiglottis (epi-GLOHT-ihs) a part of the larynx that consists of a leaf-shaped piece of hyaline cartilage which forms a movable lid over the opening into the trachea, called the glottis.

epiglottis: Gk. epi = upon, and glottis = larynx, hence the uppermost part of the larynx.

Epimysium (epi'-MI-see-uhm) the outer layer of CT associated with muscle, it surrounds the whole muscle (see deep fascia).

epimysium: Gk. epi = upon, and mys = muscle; the CT surrounding an entire muscle.

Epineurium (epi-NEW-ree-uhm) the outermost layer of CT associated with a nerve. It surrounds the whole nerve.

Epiphyseal (epi-FIS-EE-al) **line** a line of calcified bone visible in a section through bone that is the remnant of the epiphyseal plate.

Epiphyseal plate a region of cartilage b/n the epiphysis & diaphysis producing growth in the length of a bone.

Epiphysis (ep-IF-ih-sihs) the end of a long bone that contains spongy bone tissue, surrounded by compact bone.

epiphysis: Gk. epi = upon, & physis = growth, the end of a long bone beyond the cartilaginous growth disc, adj.- epiphysial.

epiploic: adj.Gk. epiploon = a net, which the greater omentum resembles (+ entrapped fat globules).

episi- to do with the vulva (ep-ee-zee)

Epithelial (epi-THEE-lee-al) **tissue** one of 3 primary tissue types, it is characterized by a close arrangement of cells with little intercellular material. (noun = epithelium, pl epithelia). Comes in various arrangements, single layered, columnar, cuboidal, pseudostratified, squamos, mutilated & stratified.

epithelium: Gk. epi = upon, & thele = the nipple; cell layer lining the body's internal & external surfaces. Epithelium of the gastrointestinal and respiratory tracts.

Eponychium (ehp'-o-NIHK-ee-uhm) a narrow region of stratum corneum at the proximal end of a nail. (= cuticle).

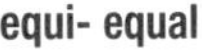

equi- equal

erector: Lt. erectus = straight or upright.

erg- work

-ergy – action

erigentes: pl., Lt. erigere = to erect.

Erysipelas (er-ee-sip-EL-us) Gk. eryth = red , pellas = skin – red, brawny skin due to infection generally streptococci along with constitutional symptoms.

erythr- red

erythema (eh-REE-thee-muh) Gk.: flushing on the skin - redness

Erythrocyte (eh-RITH-ro-site) a synonym for red blood cell.

eso- within

Esophagus (eh-SOHF-ah-guhs) a tubular segment of the alimentary canal b/n the pharynx & the stomach. (AS Oesophagus).

ethmoid: adj.Gk. ethmos = sieve, and eidos = shape or form, hence, like a sieve; an unpaired skull bone.

eu- good, normal, well, easily

eury- broad, wide

eversion: Lt. e = out, and versum = turned, hence turned outwards.

ex- to protrude, outside, out, over, away, less

Excoriation (EX-kor-ree-ay-shon) skin defect which only involves the epithelial layer see also Ulcer

Excretion (ehk-SKREE-shuhn) the process by which metabolic waste materials are removed from a cell, a tissue, or an entire body.

Exfoliation (EX-foh-lee-ay-shon) scrapping off of the outer skin layers – generally for cosmetic purposes see also Desquammation

exo- outside, outer layer, out of

Exocrine (EHK-so-krihn) gland, one of two main categories of glands, here the cellular products are released into ducts then transported to a body surface or into a body cavity.

Exocytosis (ehk'-so-sih-TO-sihs) the active cellular process by which materials are transported out of a cell and into the extracellular environment.

exogen Gk exo = out hair growth phase where the hair is shed

exophthalmos: Gk. exo = out, and ophthalmos = eye, hence, prominent eyeball.

extend: Lt. extendo = extend/stretch out, extension = extended or straightened; $\neq$ flexed or bent.

external: adj. Lt. externus = outward, hence, further from the inside.

External auditory canal the epidermal-lined tube of the external ear, extending from the auricle to the tympanic membrane. It passes through the hole in the temporal bone called the external auditory meatus.

External ear the outer part of the ear, which consists of the appendage known as the auricle, the external auditory canal, and the tympanic membrane (see Pinna).

extra- outside of, out, over, beyond, in addition to,

Extracellular environment (EKS-trah-CEHL-yew-lar en-VI-ROH-mehnt) the body space outside the plasma membrane of cells.

Extracellular fluid (**ECF**) the fluid outside the plasma membrane of cells, including interstitial fluid and blood plasma.

extraperitoneal: adj.Lt. extra = outside, Gk. peri = around and teinein = stretched, outside the serous membrane stretched around the inside of the abdominal wall and around the viscera.

extrapyramidal: Lt. extra = outside, and pyramidal (q.v.), hence descending nerve tracts that do not traverse the pyramids of the medulla.

extrinsic: Lt. extrinsecus = from without, hence (usually) a muscle (usually) originating outside the part on which it acts.

A B C D E F G H I J K L M N O P Q R S T U V W X Y Z

F

fabella: diminutive of Lt. faba = a bean, a sesamoid bone found in the lateral head of gastrocnemius.

Facet (FAS-set) a small joint surface or smooth boney surface.

facet: Lt. facies = face, a small smooth bony surface, ± coated with articular/joint cartilage, the site of a tendinous attachment (c.f. a facet on a diamond).

faci- to do with the face (fasi)

facilitate: Lt. facilis = easy, hence, to make easy.

falciform: adj.Lt. falx = a sickle, and forma = form, hence, shaped like a sickle.

Falx (FALKs) as in sickle-shaped or curved used in the brain mainly, adj. falciform (FALS-ee-form).

falx: Lt. = sickle, hence, the sickle-shaped falx cerebri and falx cerebelli, adj.- falciform.

fasci- band, connection (fashi-)

Fascia (FASH-ee-ah) a sheet or band of dense CT that structurally supports organs and tissues. Deep fascia surrounds muscle tightly, and superficial fascia separates the skin and muscle layers often loose, variable.

fascia: Lt. = band or bandage, hence the fibrous wrapping of muscles - deep fascia, or the subcutaneous layer of fatty CT - superficial fascia, adj. fascial.

Fascicle (FAS-ih-kul) A bundle of skeletal muscle fibres (cells) that forms a part of a muscle.

fasciculus: diminutive of Lt. fascis = bundle, hence, a bundle of nerve or muscle fibres.

Fat a lipid compound formed from one molecule of glycerol and three molecules of fatty acids. It is the body's most concentrated form of energy, and also serves to insulate from external temperature changes. It is stored w/n cells comprising adipose tissue.

fauces: Lt. = throat, adj.- faucial.

febri- fever

Fecalith (FEE-ku-lith) "fecal stone" – concentration of material in the intestine around fecal material AS Faeces / Faecalith.

femur: Lt. = thigh, adj.- femoral. pl. femora

fenestra: Lt. = window.

Fetus (FEE-tuhs) the early developmental stage from 8 weeks after fertilization to birth. (AS Foetus).

fetus: the developing mammal in utero; in man, after the 2nd month in utero, adj.- foetal or fetal.

fibre: Lt. fibra = a fibre, adj. Lt. fibrosus = fibrous.

fibril: diminutive of Lt. fibra = a fibre.

Fibrin (FI-brihn) an insoluble protein in the blood, formed from fibrinogen & required for blood clotting.

Fibrinogen (fi-BRIHN-o-jehn) a large plasma protein, the precursor of fibrin. It is converted to fibrin by thrombin.

Fibroblast (FI-bro-blahst) a large cell in CT that manufactures much of the extracellular material.

Fibrocartilage a type of cartilage (CT), which is distinguished from other cartilages by the small size and numbers of chondrocytes and lacunae, differential staining, and close resemblance to dense regular CT. It is found in the intervertebral discs particularly the outer ring.

"Fibroid" slang term for fibroleiomyoma – benign proliferation of smooth muscle in the uterus.

Fibrous tunic the outer wall of the eyeball that is composed of dense CT, it contains the sclera & the cornea.

fibula: Lt. = brooch, which the tibia and fibula resemble, the fibula is the movable pin.

fila- threadlike thread

filament: Lt. filamentum = a delicate fibre, adj.- filamentous.

filum: Lt. = a thread. Filum terminale - a thread of pia continuous with the lower end of the SC.

fimbria: Lt. = a fringe, fimbria hippocampi, a scalloped band of fibres alongside the hippocampus.

Fissure (FISH-er) a narrow gap or slit or furrow generally referring to a gap in the epidermis.

fissure: Lt. = a cleft.

Fistula (FIST-you-lu) Lt. tube – an abnormal opening connecting the inside of an organ to the surface of another - commonly in the female pelvis connecting the bladder and vagina (Utherovaginal) or the vagina and rectum (Rectovaginal).

fixator: Lt. fixus = fixed, hence, a muscle which fixes a part.

flaccid: adj.Lt. flaccidus = weak or slack.

flavum: adj.Lt. flavus = yellow.

flex: Lt. flexum = bent, flexor, a muscle which bends a part of the body, & flexion = the act of flexing ≠ extension.

Flagellum (flaw-JEHL-uhm) a single, long extension of a cell composed of protein filaments to provide mobility. In human cells, it is found only in sperm cells.

flav- yellow

flexure: Lt. flexura = a bending.

flocculus: diminutive of Lt. floccus, a tuft. Resembling a picture of a little cloud, with a woolly top and a flat base, as in flocculus cerebelli.

Foetus (FEE-tuhs) the early developmental stage from 8 weeks after fertilization to birth. (AS Fetus).

foetus: the developing mammal in utero; in man, after the 2nd month in utero, adj.- foetal AS fetal.

folia: plural of Lt. folium = leaf.

follicle: Lt. folliculus = a little bag, adj.- follicular.

fontanelle: French diminutive of Lt. fons = fountain, associated with the palpable pulsation of the brain in the anterior fontanelle of an infant.

Foramen (FOR-ay-men) a natural hole or passage in a bone usually for the transmission of BVs or Ns.

foramen: Lt. = hole. pl. foramina.

forceps: Lt. = tongs.

fore- front or before

forearm: the upper limb between the elbow and the wrist.

fornix: Lt. = arch (hence fornication, because the Roman prostitutes plied their profession beneath the arches of the bridges over the River Tiber).

Fossa (FOS-ah) a pit, depression or concavity on a bone or formed by several bones.

fossa: Lt. = a ditch or trench, hence a concavity in bone, or an organ, or on a lining surface.

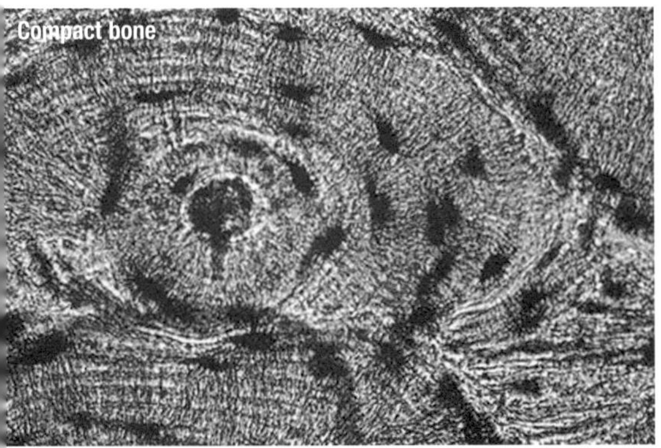
Compact bone

fovea: Lt. = a pit (usually smaller than a fossa).

Fovea centralis (FO-vee-aw cehn-TRAL-ihs) the region of the retina consisting of cone cells only (no rod cells), it is the area of highest visual acuity (sharpness of vision) a small depression on the retina.

foveola: diminutive of fovea.

fract- break

frenulum: diminutive of frenum.

frenum: Lt. = bridle or curb.

frontal: adj. Lt. frontis = of the forehead, or coronal.

Frontal plane a plane that extends in a vertical direction dividing the human body into front (anterior) and back (posterior) portions. (also = the coronal plane).

Fundus a large, expanded compartment w/n the stomach serving as a temporary storage area for ingested food material.

fundus: Lt. = bottom or base. (note that the fundus of the stomach & uterus are at the top, and the fundus of the eye & of the bladder are posterior!). adj.fundiform.

funiculus: diminutive of Lt. funis = cord (used usually for bundles of nerve fibres).

Furuncle (Fah-RUNG-kl) Lt. funuculus = petty thief description of the complexion of many thieves = the common boil, nodular pyogenic infection of the hair follicle

fus- spindle (fewze-)

fusiform: adj.Lt. fusus = spindle, hence, spindle-shaped.

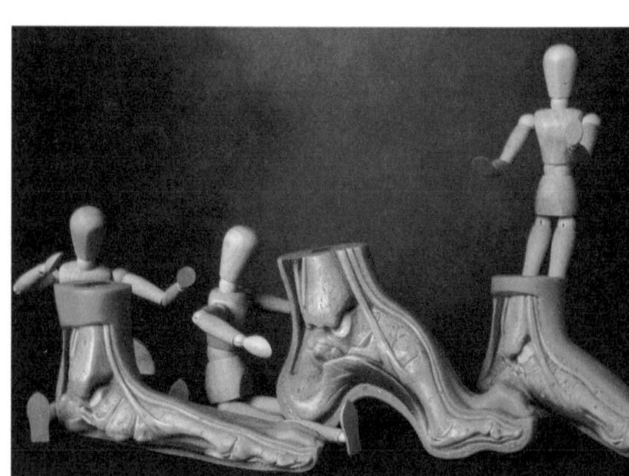

G

A B C D E F G H I J K L M N O P Q R S T U V W X Y Z

Gallbladder (GAWL-blahd-er) a small saclike organ located beneath the liver that stores bile.

galli: genetive (possessive case) of Lt. = cock, hence, crista galli, the cock's comb.

gallus: Lt. = cock, hence, crista galli, the cock's comb.

Gamete (ga-MEET) a sex cell. It may be male (sperm cell) or female (oocyte).

gamma: the 3rd letter of the Gk. alphabet, used in sequence - alpha, beta, gamma, delta, etc.

Ganglion (GANG-lee-ohn) a cluster of neuron cell bodies located outside the CNS.

ganglion: Gk. = swelling, referring to a peripheral collection of nerve cells, adj.- ganglionic.

Gastric (GAHS-trihk) **gland** any one of several types of glands in the stomach mucosa that contributes to the gastric juice.

gastric: Gk. gaster = belly or stomach adj. gastro.

Gastro (GAS-troh) pertaining to the stomach.

Gastrocnemius (GAS-troc-neem-uhs) the muscle belly in the calf.

gastrocnemius: Gk. gaster = belly, and kneme = leg, hence, the bulging muscle of the calf. gelatus = frozen.

gelatin: Lt. gelatina = congeal material derived from partial hydrolysis of skin collagen.

gemellus: Lt. diminutive of geminus = twin.

Gene (JEEN) functional unit of heritary occupying a specific place on a chromosome, which directs the formation of a specific protein.

genial: adj.Gk. geneion = chin.

geniculate: Lt. geniculare = to flex the knee, hence, a bent knee.

geniculum: Lt. geniculare = (jen-ew) the knee.

genital: adj.Lt. genitalis = reproductive, hence, genitalia, the sexual organs.

genu: Lt. = knee.

Germinal (JER-mih-nal) **epithelium** a layer of epithelial cells covering the ovaries.

Gestation (jehs-TA-shuhn) the period of development prior to birth.

gestation: Gk. ges = carry

giganto- huge

gingiva: Lt. = gum (of tooth).

girdle: a ring of bones which may be complete or incomplete

A B C D E F **G** H I J K L M N O P Q R S T U V W X Y Z

hence the pelvic girdle is complete and the pectoral girdle is not.

glabella: diminutive of Lt. glaber = bald, i.e. smooth, bony prominence between the eyebrows.

gladiolus: diminutive of L. gladius = a sword, i.e. a small sword, applied to the body of the sternum.

Gland a specialization of epithelial tissue to secrete substances. It may consist of a single cell or a multicellular arrangement.

gland: Lt. glans = an acorn, adj.- glandular; a secreting organ.

glandula: diminutive of Lt. glans = acorn, hence a little gland.

Glandular epithelium epithelial tissue whose primary function is secretion; it is the prominent tissue forming endocrine & exocrine glands.

glans: Lt. = acorn. glans penis at the end of the penis - looks like an acorn.

Glaucoma (GLAW-kohm-u) Gk:glaukoma = opacity - hence opaque colour of the crystalline lens, gp of diseases all with ↑ intraocular pressure and typical visual defects resulting from this.

glenoid: adj.Gk. glene = socket, and eidos = shape or form.

glia: Gk. = glue, hence, an adhesive CT.

globus: Lt. = a globe.

Glomerulus (glo-MEHR-oo-luhs) one of many specialized capillary networks located in the kidney cortex, each of which is encapsulated by a Bowman's capsule. It is part of the kidney nephron, & is the site of kidney filtration.

glomerulus: Lt. glomerare = to roll up, from glomus = a ball of thread (c.f. conglomeration) or knot.

glossal: adj.Gk. glossa = tongue.

glottic: adj.Gk. = larynx.

glottis: Gk. = larynx, hence, the boundaries of rima glottidis.

Gluteal (GLOO-tee-al) to do with the rump buttock behind adj. gluteus (GLOO-tee-us).

gluteal: adj.Gk. gloutos = rump or buttock.

gluteus: Gk. gluteos = rump or buttock. 1of 3 muscles of the buttock, adj. - gluteal.

gnath- jaw (na-th)

Goblet cell a unicellular gland often in the shape of a goblet that secretes mucus. (also = a mucus cell).

Golgi apparatus (GOL-jee ahp'-ah-RAHT-uhs) a cellular organelle characterized by a series of flattened, hollow cisternae. It serves as a site of anabolic activities.

Gomphosis (GOM-foh-sis) joint b/n root of a tooth and jaw bone.

Gonad (GO-nahd) an organ that produces gametes and sex H. In the male it is the testes, and in the female it is the ovaries.

Goiter (GOY-te) Lt. guttur = throat, chronic non-cancerous enlargement of the thyroid gland.

gonad: Gk. = reproduction, hence a gland producing gametes - ovary or testis, adj. - gonadal.

gon- sexual

goni- corner

gony- knee

gnos - Gk: gnos = to know (nos) agnos = not to know (AG-nos).

gonad: Gk. = reproduction, hence a gland producing gametes - ovary or testis, adj. - gonadal.

Graafian follicle: a mature ovarian follicle that contains a single oocyte. The Graafian follicle secretes the female hormone estrogen. Following ovulation, it changes form to become the corpus luteum, which produces progesterone.

gracile: adj. Lt. gracilis = slender.

Grade - in pathology refers to the extent of the cancer spread - and so the method of management.

granul- grain (gran-ewl)

granulation: diminutive of Lt. granum = a grain, hence a little grain

Granuloma (GRAN-you-loh-mu) -nodular granular lesions of inflammation - granulomatosis - process of forming these inflammatory nodules, generally containing epitheloid cells & monocytes in a fibrocyte stroma.

gravid: adj. Lt. gravida = pregnant.

gravis- heavy

Grey matter Nerve tissue in the brain and SC that contains neuron cell bodies, dendrites, & nonmyelinated axons, and therefore appears grey or non-white in colour.

griseum: adj. Lt. griseus = bluish or pearly grey.

gubernaculum: Lt. something which governs or directs, like a rudder (c.f. gubernatorial).

Gustation (guhs-TA-shuhn) the sense of taste.

gustatory: adj. Lt. gustatio = taste, hence, pertaining to the sense of taste.

Gustatory organ: a special sensory organ that contains chemoreceptors providing the sense of taste, or gustation. (also = taste buds) They are mainly located on the tongue & embedded w/n papillae.

Gyrus (g-eye-rus) the elevation of neural tissue in the brain, opposite of sulcus the depression in the brain b/n each gyri.

gyrus: Gk. gyros = circle, hence a coil of brain cortex. pl. gyri.

gymno- nakedness

gyn- female (g-eye-n)

A B C D E F H H I J K L M N O P Q R S T U V W X Y Z

H

habenula: diminutive of Lt. habena = rein.

Haeme = blood (AS Heme).

Haematocrit (hee-MAT-o-krit) the percentage of RBCs in a sample of blood, which is determined by centrifuging the sample and measuring the RBC volume relative to other blood components.

Haematopoiesis (heem'-ah-to-poy-EE-sihs) The production of blood cells in the red bone marrow. (= haemopoiesis. AS hematopoiesis).

Haemoglobin (HEE-mo-glo-bihn) a complex protein in RBCs involved in the transport of oxygen & carbon dioxide. (AS hemoglobin).

Haemolysis (hee-MOL-ih-sihs) the bursting of a RBC resulting from disruption of the plasma membrane by toxins, freezing or thawing, or exposure to a hypotonic solution. (AS hemolysis).

Haemorrhage (HEM-or-ayj) GK. haeme = blood, rhegnymi = to burst forth, hence loss of blood outside the CVS.

Haemostasis (hee'-mo-STA-sihs) the stoppage of bleeding.

haemorrhoid: Gk. haema = blood, & rheo = to flow, hence likely to bleed, hence haemorrhoids are the extrusion of gut BVs through the anus. These have little or no muscle and so bleeding can be profuse.

Hair a threadlike outgrowth of the skin that is composed of columns of keratinized cells.

Hair follicle a cluster of epithelial tissue surrounding the root of a hair where the hair originates.

hallux- big toe (hal-uhcs)

hallux: Lt. hallex = great toe (hallucis = of the great toe).

Hamartoma (ham-ar-TOE-mar) bodily defect causing an overgrowth of tissue - not cancerous.

hamate: adj. Lt. hamus = a hook, hence, hooked.

hamstrings: the tendons of the muscles of the ham - ie. of the back of the thigh - felt behind the knee when the leg is flexed against resistance (semimembranosus, semitendinosus and biceps femoris).

hamulus: diminutive of Lt. hamus = hook.

hapl- single

haustra: Lt. = saccules.

Haversian system (see osteon) smallest functioning unit of bone.

Heart the hollow muscular organ within the thoracic cavity that propels blood through the circulatory network.

A B C D E F G **H** I J K L M N O P Q R S T U V W X Y Z

hecl- ulcer (hels)

helicine: Gk. helix = a coil, spiral.

helix: Gk. = coil.

heme see haeme.

hemi- half (hem-ee)

hemianopia: Gk. hemi = half, an = negative, opsis = vision, hence loss of half of the field of vision.

hemianopsia: Gk. hemi = half, an = negative, opsis = vision, hence loss of half of the field of vision.

hemiparesis: Gk. hemi = half, paresis = paralysis, used usually to denote weakness rather than paralysis.

hemiplegia: Gk. hemi = half, plegia = stroke, hence, paralysis of one half of the body.

hemisphere: Gk. hemi = half, sphaira = ball, hence, half of a sphere

hepar: Gk. = liver, adj.- hepatic.

Hepatic (heh-PAT-ik) pertaining to the liver.

hepatic: adj.Gk. hepar = the liver.

Hepatocytes (heh-PAT-OH-cites) Liver cells.

hernia: Lt. = a protrusion, adj.- hernial.

heter- other, different, abnormal ≠ homo

hex- six

hiatus: Lt. = a gap (like that between some people's ears).

hidr- sweat

Hidrosis (HEYE-droh-sis) disease of the sweat glands.

hier- to do with the sacrum

hilum: Lt. = the point of attachment of a seed, hence the part of an organ where the vessels and nerves are attached; adj.-hilar.

hindbrain: the part of the brain below tentorium cerebelli, i.e. medulla oblongata + pons + cerebellum.

hip: the lateral prominence of the hip bone & greater trochanter.

hippocampus: Gk. hippokampos = a sea-horse, the curled shape of the hippocampus in coronal section

hippus (Gk. hippos = horse) fluctuation of the pupil under steady illumination

hist- tissues

Histology (HIHS-toh-lo-jee) the microscopic study of tissues.

histology Lt. = pictures, ology = the study of, hence the study of pictures

Horizontal plane a plane that extends perpendicular to the length of the body dividing it into superior and inferior portions. (also = transverse plane).

holo- entire

homo- same (hoh-moh)

homeo- same, common, like (hoh-me-oh)

homologous: adj. Gk. homos = same, & logos = word, parts with similar morphologies but different functions.

horizontal: adj.- parallel to the horizon.

Hordeolum (Hord-ee-oh-lum) Lt = barley grain – a small pustule on the eyelid = stye.

horm- to urge, to stimulate

Hormone (HOR-mone) a substance secreted by endocrine tissue that changes the physiological activity of the target cell.

horn: a projection, often pointed.

humer- to do with the arm, upper arm (hew-mer)

humerus: Lt. = the arm-bone.

humour: Lt. humor = liquid, hence the aqueous & vitreous humour of the eyeball.

hyal- glass

hyaline: adj.Gk. hyalos = glassy.

Hyaline cartilage (HY-al-ine) a type of CT that contains chondrocytes embedded w/n lacunae, both of which are surrounded by a dense, semitranslucent matrix of collagen fibres &

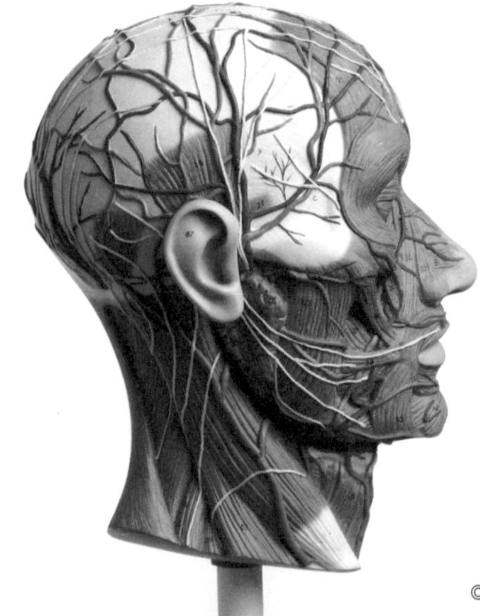

glycosaminoglycans. Hyaline cartilage is found in: tracheal & bronchial walls, the costal cartilages, the nose, the endos of all syovial joints & the larynx.

hydr- water

hydrocephalus: Gk. hydor = water, koilos = head. (c.f. cephalic).

hydrops = oedema

hygr- water

hymen: Gk. = membrane; across the virginal vagina.

hyoid: adj.Gk. = U-shaped.

hyper - excessive ≠ hypo

hyperacusis: Gk. hyper = over, and akousis = hearing, hence excessive sensitivity to sound.

hypoglossal: adj. Gk. hypo = under, and glossa = tongue.

Hyperplasia (HI'-per-PLAY-zee-ah) an increased production & growth of cells beyond normal limits.

Hypertonic (HI'-pehr-TOHN-ihk) the state of a solution having a greater concentration of dissolved particles than the solution it is compared to (≠ hypotonic).

Hypertrophy (hi'-PEHR-tro-fee) the abnormal enlargement or growth of a cell, tissue, or organ.

hypo- deficient, below, under ≠ hyper

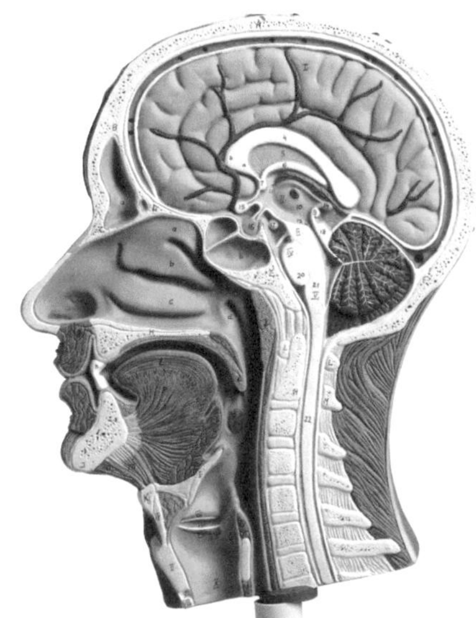

Hypodermis (hi'-po-DEHRM-ihs) the area of the body b/n the dermis of the skin and skeletal muscle

Hyponychium thickened epidermis which forms the floor of the nail fold to the undersurface of the nail see also Subungual.

> hypophysis: Gk. hypo = down, physis = growth, hence, a downgrowth (from the brain). However, this is not the whole truth. Part of this gland is an upgrowth from the pharynx, adj.- hypophysial. (=pituitary).

Hyposecretion (hi'-po-see-KREE-shuhn) the diminished secretion of a product by a gland.

Hypothalamus (hi'-po-THAHL-aw-muhs) the small, inferior portion of the diencephalon in the brain. It functions mainly in the control of involuntary activities, including endocrine gland regulation, sleep, thirst & hunger.

> hypothalamus: Gk. hypo = under, and thalamus (q.v.), refers to part of diencephalon.

Hypotonic (hi'-po-TON-ik) the state of a solution having a lower concentration of dissolved particles that the solution it is compared to (≠ hypertonic).

hyster- uterine (hister-)

> hystero: Gk. hyster = to do with the uterus thought to be the seat of all female emotion, hence adj.- hysterical pertains to female emotions- over exhibitionistic emotion, noun. hysteria.

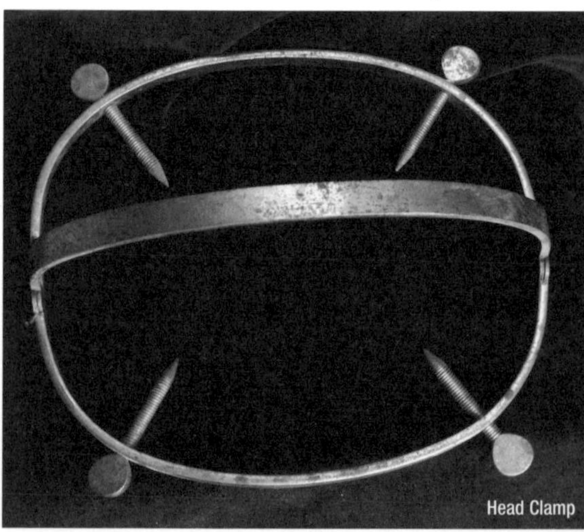

Head Clamp

I

iatr- to treat (ee-at-rah)
ictero- jaundiced
ichthy. Gk. = fish
Ichthyosis (IK-thee-oh-sis) generalized term for any skin disease characterized by any increased or aberrant keratinization of the skin – gish skin
idio- one's own, separate, unknown
Idiopathic (ID-ee-oh-path- ic) unknown
idiopathic: Gk.=idios=one's self, pathos=sickness-a spontaneous sickness or illness of unknown origin = agnogenic.
icter- jaundice (ikter)
ile- pertaining to the ileum
Ileum (IHL-ee-uhm) the distal segment of the small intestine.
ileum: Gk. eilein = twisted. adj.- ileal.
ili- pertaining to the flank or the leg
ilium: Lt. the bone of the flank, adj.- iliac.
im- in, into, on, onto, not, non
ima: adj. Lt. = lowest, hence artery thyroidea ima lowest artery to the thyroid.
impacted Lt. impacto = to strike against, hence wedged, closely packed & so immovable, generally referring to teeth imprisoned in the alveolus.
impar: Lt. = unpaired.
in- in, into, on, onto, not, non
In vitro (ihn VEE-tro) outside the body, such as in a culture bottle.
In vivo (ihn VEE-vo) inside the living body.
incisor: Lt. incisum = cut up.
incisura: Lt. = notch.
incus: Lt. = anvil, hence the anvil-shaped ossicle of the middle ear.
index: Lt. = a pointer, hence, the fore-finger. adj. indicis
indusium: Lt. = tunic.
infarct Lt. infarctus = to stuff into, hence the wedge shape of dead tissue resulting from a sudden insufficiency in the arteriole BS.
infero- low, lower
Inferior (ihn-FER-ee-or) a directional term describing a location further from the head than something else.
inferior: adj.Lt. = lower down, hence, farther from the head end.
Inflammation (in-FLAM-ay-shon) body response to any irritation.

A B C D E F G H I J K L M N O P Q R S T U V W X Y Z

infra- below, beneath

infra: Lt. = below.

Infundibulum (ihn'-fuhn-DIB-yoo-lum) the narrow connection b/n the hypothalamus of the brain & the pituitary gland, also, the funnel-shaped distal end of the uterine tube which opens near an ovary.

infundibulum: Lt. = funnel & the fluid opening in the Left ventricle.

inguin- pertaining to the groin

inguinal: adj.Lt. inguen = groin.

inhibition: Lt. inhibitus = restrained, hence, reduction of the excitability of a synapse.

innervate: Lt. in = into, and nervus = nerve, hence, to supply a nerve to a part.

innominate: Lt. in = not, and nomen = name, hence, without a name, hence innominate bone = unnamed bone generally referring to the hip.

insert: Lt. insertio = to join into, implant, hence, to attach; noun insertion.

inspection: Lt. inspectus = examined, hence, visual examination.

insul- island

insula: Lt. = island.

Integumentary (ihn-tehg'-yoo-MEHN-tar-ee) pertaining to the skin & its accessory organs.

integument: Lt. in = on, tegmen = roof, hence the skin coat.

inter- between

intercalated: adj. Lt. inter = between, and calatum = inserted, hence interposed.

Intercalated disk (ihn-ter'-kaw-LA-ted dihsk) a transverse thickening of a cardiac muscle cell's sarcolemma at its boundary with an adjacent cell. It aids in the conduction of an impulse from one cardiac cell to another.

Intercellular (ihn'-tehr-SEHL-yoo-lar) the area b/n cells.

interdigitate: Lt. inter = between, and digitus = a digit, hence, to interlock - like fingers.

Internal (ihn-TER-nawl) a directional term describing a location deep to the surface of the skin relative to something else.

internal: adj. Lt. internus = inward, hence, nearer the inside.

interstitial: adj. Lt. inter = between, & sistum = set, hence, set between.

Interstitial cells (ihn'-ter-STIH-shuhl) cells in the testes located b/n seminiferous tubules that secrete testosterone. (= cells of Leydig).

Interstitial fluid (ihn'-tehr-STIH-shuhl FLOO-ihd) the portion of extracellular fluid which fills the tissue spaces b/n cells. (= tissue fluid and intercellular fluid).

Intervertebral disk (ihn'-tehr-VEHR-teh-brahl disk) a cartilaginous joint consisting of a pad of fibrocartilage located b/n two adjacent vertebrae.

Intestinal gland (ihn-TEHS-tihn-awl glahnd) a tubular gland in the mucosa of the small intestine which secretes digestive enzymes. (= crypt of Leiberkuhn).

intestine: Lt. intestinum = the digestive tube beyond the stomach.

intima: Lt. = innermost.

intra- within

intra: Lt. = within.

Intracellular (ihn'-traw-SEHL-yoo-lar) the space w/n a cell ≠ intercellular fluid ≠ extracellular fluid.

Intracellular fluid (**ICF**) the fluid w/n cells.

intrafusal: adj. Lt. intra = within, fusus = spindle.

Intramembranous ossification (ihn'-trah-MEHM-braw-nuhs ohs'-ih-fih-KA-shuhn) the development of bone from foetal CT membranes.

intrinsic: adj. Lt. = on the inside.

introitus: Lt. intro = within, and ire = to go, i.e. an orifice or point of entry to a cavity or space.

inversion: Lt. = in, and vertere = to turn, hence to turn inward, inside out, upside down.

ipsi- same

ipsilateral: Lt. ipsi = self, the same, and latus = side, hence on the same side ≠ contralateral.

Iris (I-rihs) a part of the vascular tunic of the eye. It is located on the anterior side of the eyeball & is composed of smooth muscle fibres that regulate the amount of light entering the eye. The iris is the coloured part of the eye surrounding the pupil.

iris: Lt. = a rainbow.

isch- suppression, blocking

Ischaemia (is-KEEM-ee-ya) result of sudden decrease in the BS to cells or tissues

ischi- hip

ischium: Gk. ischion = socket, because the ischium contributes more than either the ilium or pubis to the acetabulum.

Islet of Langerhans (I-leht of LANG-er-hawnz) one of numerous clusters of endocrine cells w/n the pancreas.

iso- equal, similar

iso: Gk. = equal.

Isotonic solution a solution that contains an equal amount of solutes relative to another.

isthmus: Gk. isthmos - a narrow passage.

J

Jejunum (jeh-JEW-nuhm) the middle segment of the small intestine.
jejunum: Lt. jejunus = empty, adj.- jejunal.

Joint (joynt) a point of contact b/n two opposing bones, which may move. (also = articulation).
joint: the meeting of 2 or more bones or cartilages, at which movement is possible.

jug- yoke (jug)

jugu- throat (jug-ew)
jugular: adj.Lt. jugulum = neck.

Jugum (JOO-gum) referring to the bridge b/n 2 bones generally symmetrical with a Right and Left side (pl. juga).
jugum: Lt. = yoke (cf. conjugal).

juxta- near to
juxta: Lt. = near. next to

Juxtaglomerular apparatus (juhks'-tah-glo-MER-yoo-lawr ahp'-ah-RAHT-uhs) a structure located in a kidney nephron which is composed of cells from the distal convoluted tubule & the afferent arteriole. It secretes renin in response to a decrease in BP.

K

kary- nucleus
kel- tumor
Keloid (KEE-loyd) - skin tumor - overgrowth of skin and scar tissue particularly as the result of injury / surgery
kerato- horny, hard, skin, cornea
Keratin (KER-ah-tihn) a waterproofing protein present in the epidermis, nails, and hair.

keratin: Gk. keras = horn.

kine- move
-kines stimulation of activation for division or growth of cells

kinocilium: Gk. kineo = to move (cf. kinetic), and cilium Lt. = eyelash, hence protoplasmic thread of hair process in cupula of crista ampullaris of a semicircular duct.

knee: the junction of the thigh and the leg. (see genu = knee).

koilo- hollow concave
kolp- vagina

koniocortex: Gk. konis = dust, and Lt. cortex = bark, hence, sensory cortex containing mostly granular layers.

kyphosis: Gk. kyphos = bent or bowed forward.

L

labi- lip

labium: Lt. = lip (plural labia), adj.- labial.
labrum: Lt. = rim.
labyrinth: Gk. labyrinthos = maze, adj.- labyrinthine.
lacerum: Lt. lacer = mangled, hence, lacerated, tornforamen lacerum is often torn in head injuries.

lacri- tear (lak-ree)

lacrimal: adj. Lt. lacrima = a tear (drop).
lactation: Lt. lactans = suckling. Hence, the act of secreting milk.

Lacteal =lactiferous ducts, specialized lymphatic ducts in the small intestine to absorb large fat molecules. When they do so they turn pale or milky.

lacteal: adj. Lt. lac = milk, hence, resembling milk.
lactic: adj. Lt. lac = milk.
lactiferous: adj. Lt. lac = milk, and ferre = to carry.

Lacuna (lah-KOO-nah) a chamber w/n bone or cartilage matrix which houses a cell (an osteocyte or chondrocyte). pl. - lacunae.

lacuna: Lt. lacus = lake, hence, a small pond or gap, adj.lacunar.

lal- talking

lambda: Gk. letter representing a capital 'L' and written as an inverted V. adj. lambdoid (L-shaped).

Lamella (lah-MEHL-uh) concentric ring of hardened bone matrix found in compact bone. pl. lamellae.

lamella: diminutive of Lt. lamina = plate; hence, a small plate.

Lamina (lah-MIN-uh) plate as in the lamina of the vertebra a plate of bone connecting the vertical and transverse spines pl. laminae (lah-MIN-ee) laminectomy = removal of the lamina to give access to the SC and its perforating nerves.

lamina: Lt. = plate, either a layer of NT, like the laminae of the lateral geniculate body, or a CT membrane, like lamina cribrosa sclerae, or of bone, as in vertebral laminae; laminectomy = lamina + Gk. ektome = excision - excision of the vertebral laminae, adj.- aminar.
lanugo: Lt. lana = wool, the fine downy hair on the skin of the foetus, or cheeks or malnutrition.

lapar- abdominal cavity
lapis- stone

Large intestine the final segment of the alimentary canal consisting of a large tube that forms the faeces, which is expelled by the process of defecation.

Larynx (LAR-ihnks) a box-like cartilaginous organ in the respiratory tract located b/n the pharynx & the trachea.

larynx: Gk. = voice-box, adj.- laryngeal.

lata: Lt. latus = side.

Lateral (LA-tehr-awl) a directional term describing a structure that is located further from the vertical midline of the body relative to another.

lateral: adj. Lt. latus = side, hence, nearer the side.

latissimus: superlative of adj.Lt. latus = wide, hence, latissimus dorsi muscle, the widest muscle of the back; earlier name was anitersor - wiper of the anus.

leg: the lower limb b/n the knee & the ankle.

leio- smooth

lemniscus: Gk. lemniskos = a band or ribbon (applied to nerve fibres).

Lens an oval, transparent structure located b/n the posterior iris & the vitreous humor of the eyeball. It is connected to the vascular tunic by suspensory ligaments -it is a cataract if it becomes opaque.

lens: Lt. = lentil - transparent body with surfaces curved to re-direct light adj. lentiform or lenticular.

lentiform: adj.Lt. lens = lentil, & forma = shape, hence, lentil- shaped.

lentigo Lt. freckle – brown / tan spot on the skin.

lepto- thin, delicate small mild

leptomeninx: Gk. lepto = delicate, & meninx = membrane.

Lesion (LEE-zshen) a destructive change in the tissue - such as an inflammation, injury or wound. Generally refers to pia & arachnoid meninges.

leuco- white, colourless, pale (AS leuko)

leuko- white, colourless, pale (AS leuco)

Leucocyte (LOO-ko-site) a white blood cell. (AS leukocyte).

Leukocyte (LOO-ko-site) a white blood cell. (AS leucocyte).

levator- to lift up ≠ depressor

levator: Lt. = elevator. ≠ depressor

lien- spleen (leen)

lien: Lt. = spleen, adj.- lienal.

levo- left

liga- bind

Ligament (LIHG-ar-ment) a band or cord of dense CT that extends from one bone to another to provide a joint with structural stability.

A B C D E F G H I J K **L** M N O P Q R S T U V W X Y Z

ligament: Lt. ligamentum = bandage, usually tying parts to each other, adj.- ligamentous.

limbic: adj. Lt. limbus = a margin, usually curved. limbus: Lt. = a margin, usually curved, hence, limbus of cornea, its circular junction with the sclera, adj. - limbic; the brain limbic lobe is made up of structures which encircle the junction of the diencephalon and telencephalon.

limen: Lt. = a threshold, hence, subliminal - below threshold.

linea- line (lin-ee-ah)

linea: Lt. = line.

lingu- tongue see also gloss-

lingua: Lt. = tongue, adj. lingual.

Lingual (LIHN-gwal) pertaining to the tongue. For example, the lingual frenulum connects the tongue to the floor of the mouth.

lingula: diminutive of lingua, hence, a little tongue, adj.- lingular.

lio- smooth

lip- fat

Lipid (LIH-pihd) an organic compound that is usually insoluble in water but soluble in alcohol, ether, and chloroform. It includes fats, phospholipids, and steroids.

Lipoprotein (lih'-po-PRO-teen) a protein-lipid complex produced by the liver that transports cholesterol and triglycerides through the BS. Low density lipoproteins (LDLs) are associated with an increased risk of atherosclerosis, whereas high density lipoproteins (HDLs) are associated with a reduced risk.

lith- stone

Livedo - discoloured spot on the skin due to passive congestion.

Liver a large digestive organ in the superior right corner of the abdominopelvic cavity that functions mainly in the interconversion of energy-storage molecules, detoxification of blood, and production of bile.

livid Lt = lividus lead coloured – discolouration from a contusion or congested pooled blood.

Lobe - (LOH-b) roundish projection of any structure.

Lobules - little lobe (lob-YOOL) when pertaining to the liver, the lobules are cuboidal subdivisions of the liver that contain row upon row of hepatocytes.

lobule: diminutive of lobus.

lobulus: Lt. diminutive of lobus, hence, a lobule.

lobus: Gk. lobos = lobe, adj.- lobar.

loc- location place

locus: Lt. a place (cf. location, locate, dislocate).

loin: Lt. lumbus - the part of the back b/n the ribs & the hip bone.

longus- long

longissimus: superlative of Lt. longus = long, hence, the longest.
longitudinal: adj.Lt. longitudo = length, hence, lengthwise.
longus: adj.Lt. = long, hence, longissimus (superlative) = the longest.

Loose connective tissue a type of CT consisting of loosely-packed protein fibres of collagen and elastin in a semifluid matrix, which are produced by fibroblasts. (also = areolar tissue). It is the most widespread of all CT.

luc- light (loo-s)

lucidum: Lt. lucidus = clear.

lue- syphilis

lumb- loin

lumbar: Lt. lumbus = loin adj.- see loin.
lumbrical: Lt. lumbricus = worm, hence worm-shaped muscles of the palm.

Lumen (LOO-mehn) the potential space w/n a tubular structure. i.e. the hole in the tube.

lumen: Lt. = opening, hence the space within a tube.
lunate: adj. Lt. luna = moon, hence, crescentic.

Luncula the half moon shape at the base of the nail bed.

Lung one of two large organs in the thoracic cavity which is responsible for the exchange of respiratory gases.

lupus- (Loo-pus) Gk = wolf specifically, disease of the skin which is highly destructive and deposits collagenous lesions all over the body –looking like the skin was gnawed

luteum: adj. Lt. = yellow.

ly- dissolved

Lymph (lihmf) the slow-moving fluid w/n lymphatic vessels of the lymphatic system.

lymph: Lt. lympha - clear spring water. adj. - lymphoid, lymphatic

Lymph node a small, oval organ located w/n the lymphatic vessel network.

Lymph nodules a compact cluster of lymphocytes w/n a lymph node.

lymphatic: a vessel carrying lymph.

Lymphatic tissue a specialized type of CT containing an abundance of lymphocytes. (= lymphoid tissue).

Lymphatic vessel a hollow tubular structure similar to a vein that transports lymph in a direction leading toward the heart.

Lymphocyte (LIHM-fo-site) a type of WBC lacking large granules in the cytoplasm, it plays a central role in immunity.

lys- disintegrate

Lysosome (LI-so-sohm) a cellular organelle that contains digestive enzymes.

A B C D E F G H I J K **M** M N O P Q R S T U V W X Y Z

M

macro- big

macroscopic: adj.Gk. makros = large, & skopein = to examine; hence, large enough to be seen with the naked eye, e.g., pertaining to gross anatomy.

Macrophage (MAK-ro-fahrj) a large phagocytic cell originating from a monocyte.

macula: Lt. = spot (cf. immaculate - spotless); adj.- macular.

Macula lutea (MAK-yoo-law LOO-tee-ah) a yellow-colored depression in the retina of the eye.

Macule nonpaplapable coloured mark on the skin.

magna- large, great

makro- big

mal- abnormal bad

malac- soft

malar- cheek bone

Malignant (MAL-ig-nant) cancerous cells which invade other body parts.

magna: Lt. = great.

Major (MAY-jaw) bigger of the 2 things

malleolus: diminutive of Lt. malleus = hammer, adj.- malleolar.

Malleus (MAL-ee-uhs) the lateral ear bone that contacts the tympanic membrane; = the hammer.

malleus: Lt. = a hammer.

mamma: Lt. = breast; adj.- mammary.

Mammary (MAM-ar-ree) **gland** a modified sweat gland in the breast that serves as the gland of milk secretion for nourishment of the young.

mammilla: diminutive of mamma; adj.- mammillary.

mandible: Lt. mandere = to chew; hence, the movable lower jaw; adj.- mandibular.

manubrium: Lt. = handle; adj.- manubrial.

man- hand

manus: Lt. = hand (cf. manual).

Marrow (MAR-oh) the soft, highly vascularized tissue w/n bone. It includes yellow marrow, consisting of adipose tissue, and red marrow, which consists of blood-forming tissue. (also = haeopoietic tissue).

margin: the edge or border of a surface; adj.- marginal.

masseter: Gk. = chewer; adj.- masseteric.

mast- pertaining to the breast

Mast cell (MAH-st) a basophil that has migrated out of the BS to the extracellular tissue generally found in loose CT. It secretes heparin (an anticoagulant) and seratonin (promotes inflammation) and the immune response.

mastication: Lt. masticere = to chew.

mastoid: adj.Gk. mastos = breast or teat, and eidos = shape or form. (mass-toyd).

Matrix (MAY-trihks) the intercellular material in CT.

matrix: Lt. = a female animal used for breading, womb; refers to ground substance of CT, and nail bed.

maxilla: Lt. = jaw-bone; now used only for the upper jaw; adj.- maxillary.

maz- breast

meat- opening

Meatus (mee-AY-tus) canal, opening passage

meatus: Lt. = passage; adj.- meatal.

medi- middle, intermediate

Medial (MEE-dee-al) a directional term describing a part lying nearer to the vertical midline of the body relative to another part.

medial: adj.Lt. medius = middle; hence, nearer the median plane.

median: Lt. medianus = in the middle.

Mediastinum (mee'-dee-ah-STIH-nuhm) the region in the thoracic cavity b/n the two pleural cavities. It consists of the heart, part of the oesophagus, part of the trachea, and the major vessels of the heart.

mediastinum: Lt. medius = middle, and stans = standing; a median vertical partition, adj- mediastinal.

medius: Lt. = middle.

Medulla (meh-DUL-ah) an inner, or deeper, part of an organ. e.g. the medulla of the kidneys, the medulla of the adrenal gland & the lymph node. ≠ cortex.

medulla: Lt. = marrow; applied to part of an organ deep to its cortex; & to the SC & adjoining part of brain stem adj.- medullary.

Medulla oblongata (meh-DUHL-ah ob'-long-GAR-tah) the inferior part of the brain stem.

Medullary cavity (mehd-UL-lar-ee KAV-ih-tee) the potential space w/n the shaft of a long bone. In the adult this contains yellow marrow.

meg- large

A B C D E F G H I J K L **M** N O P Q R S T U V W X Y Z

megalo- large
meio- reduce, contract
mel- limb, cheek
melan- black

Melanin (MEHL-ah-nihn) a dark pigment released into some parts of the body like the skin.

Melanocyte (MEHL-ahn-o-site') a cell normally located deep to the epidermis in the skin that secretes melanin.

Melanoma (mehl-an-OH-mah) a highly metastatic malignancy. arising from melanocytes in the skin. (also = malignant melanoma).

Melatonin (mehl'-ah-TO-nihn) a H secreted by the pineal gland. It may play a role in circadian rhythms.

Membrane (MEHM-brane) a thin sheet of tissue that lines or covers body structures. It may contain a thin layer of epithelial tissue and CT, or only CT.

membrane: Lt. membrana = a thin sheet; adj.- membranous.

Membranous bone a type of embryonic osseous tissue representing early skeletal development in a late embryo.

men- menses

meninges: pl. of Gk. meninx = a membrane; adj.- meningeal.
meniscus: Lt. menis - a small crescent.

ment- mind, chin

mental: adj.- Lt. mentum = chin; or Lt. mens = mind.

mer- part, segment
mes- middle

mesencephalon: Gk. mesos = middle, and enkephalos = brain; adj.- mesencephalic.
mesenchyme: Gk. mesos = middle, & chymos = juice; the embryonic CT of the mesoderm.
mesentery: Gk. mesos = middle, and enteron = intestine; the peritoneal fold which tethers the centrally placed small intestine; adj. - mesenteric.

Mesoderm (MEEZ-oh-derm) the middle of the three primary germ layers in a developing embryo that forms the muscles, the heart and BVs, & the CT.

mesoderm: Gk. mesos = middle, and derma = skin; the middle germ layer of the embryo.

Mesothelium (mehz'-oh-THEE-lee-uhm) a simple squamous epithelium lining parts of the body's ventral cavity.

mesosalpinx: Gk. mesos = middle, and salpinx = tube; the

intermediate part of the broad ligament.

meta- subsequent, transformation, between, changing after

metacarpus: Gk. meta = after, & karpus = wrist; adj.- metacarpal
metachromasia: Gk. meta = after and chrome = colour; a phenomenon where different tissues are stained colours not seen in the original dye after the dye has bound to that tissue.
metaplasia Gk. meta =after plasia = growth / formation, a phenomenon where cells change their shape and properties after maturity – happens in cancerous transformation.
metaphysis: Gk. meta = after, and physis = growth; hence, b/n the 2 ends of a long bone. Alongside the epiphysial or growth cartilage; adj.- metaphysial.

Metastasis (met-AS-ta-sis) – a growth of cancerous cells in other body parts not physically linked to the primary source (V metastasize).

metatarsus: Gk. meta = after, and tarsos = ankle; hence, the bones beyond the tarsus, adj. - metatarsal.
metopic: adj.Gk. metopon = forehead.

micro- small

Microfilament (mi'-kro-FIHL-ah-mehnt) a rod-shaped component of cytoplasm composed of protein. It provides mobility for the cell.

Microglia (mi'-kro-GLEE-aw) a type of neuroglia in the brain characterized by its small size & phagocytic function.

Microtubule (mi'-kro-ew-yool) a tube-shaped component of cytoplasm composed of protein providing support & shape for the cell.

Microvilli (mi'-kro-VIHL-i) microscopic extensions of the cell membrane filled with cytoplasm that serve to increase the absorptive surface area of the cell.

micturition: Lt. micturare = to desire to pass urine.

mid- middle

Midbrain (MID-brayn) the superior part of the brain stem, located b/n the diencephalon and the pons. It serves as a relay center for impulses. (also = the mesencephalon).

Middle ear the area of the ear b/n the tympanic membrane of the outer ear & the bony labyrinth of the inner ear. It is an epithelial-lined space housing the 3 ear ossicles. (also = the tympanic cavity).

Midsagittal (MID-sahj-ih-tahl) a plane that extends vertically through the body, dividing it into unequal right and left portions.

miliary: grainlike - describing small millet seed like lesions

milli- thousandth

minimus- smallest

minimus: Lt. = smallest.

minor- smaller of 2 things

mio- reduced contraction

miosis: Gk. meiosis = lessening; hence, pupillary constriction; adj.- miotic.

Mitochondrion (mite'-o'-KOHN-dree-ohn) a cellular organelle that consists of a double layer of plasma membrane where many of the catabolic activities of the cell take place.

Mitosis (mi-TO-sihs) the division of a cell's nucleus into two daughter nuclei, each of which contains the same genetic composition as the original parent. When mitosis is followed by cytokinesis, equal division of the whole cell results.

Mixed nerve a nerve that contains axons from sensory & motor neurons.

mnem- memory (mem)

modality: Lt. modus = mode; hence, a form of sensation - e.g. touch, pain, sight.

modiolus: Lt. a cylindrical borer with a serrated edge; hence, like a screw; the central stem of the bony cochlea.

Modiolus (MOHD-ee-oh-loes) point of insewrtion of all the facial muscles around the lips.

molar: adj.Lt. mola = mill.

Monocyte (MON-oh-site) a large, agranular WBC that is phagocytic. If the cell moves from the BS to the extracellular tissue, it is called a macrophage.

mons: Lt. = mountain; mons pubis, the soft tissue bulge over the female pubes.

morph- shape

morphology: Gk. morphos = form, and logos = word or relation; hence, study of pattern of structure; adj.- morphological.

Motor end plate the portion of the sarcolemma of a muscle fibre that is in close association with a motor neuron.

Motor nerve a nerve that contains axons from motor neurons, and thereby transmits impulses away from the CNS.

Mucosa (myoo-KO-saw) an epithelial membrane that lines a body cavity or organ & contains cells that secrete mucus. (= mucous membrane).

Mucous (MYOO-kuhs) **cell** a unicellular gland that secretes mucus. (= a goblet cell).

Mucus (MYOO-kuhs) a thick fluid secretion from mucous cells, containing mostly water & polysaccharides.

multi- many (mul-tee)

multifidus: Lt. multus = much, and findere = to split.

Muscle (MUSS-l) an organ composed of skeletal muscle tissue & its associated CT that functions mainly in the production of movement of the skeleton.

muscle: Lt. musculus, diminutive of Gk. mus = mouse, the body & head of which represent the main belly of a muscle, & the tail, the tendon.

Muscle fibre a synonym for muscle cell.

Muscle tissue one of the 4 primary types of tissue in the body, characterized by its ability to contract.

Muscularis (muhs'-kyoo-LAHR-ihs) a layer of smooth muscle tissue w/n the wall of an organ.

mycet- fungal (my-seet-)

mydriasis: Gk. = dilatation of the pupil.

myc- fungal (meyec-)

myel- bone marrow, spinal cord

myelin: Gk. myelos = marrow; hence, white fatty sheath of an axis cylinder; adj. -.myelinated.

Myelin sheath (MI-eh-lihn sheth) a white, segmented insulative cover over the axons of many peripheral neurons that is produced by Schwann cells. A neuron axon that is covered by the myelin sheath is said to be myelinated.

myenteric: Gk. mys = muscle, & enteron = intestine, pertaining to the muscle of the gut.

myl- molar

mylohyoid: Gk. mylo = molar, and hyoeides = U-shaped.

Myocardium (mi'-o-KAHR-dee-uhm) the primary layer of the heart wall, composed of cardiac muscle tissue.

myocardium: Gk. mys = muscle, and kardia = heart, adj.- myocardial.

Myofibril (mi'-o-FI-brihl) a rod-shaped component of a muscle fibre, which extends the length of the fibre and is composed of thin and thick filaments of protein.

Myometrium (mi'-o-MEE-tree-uhm) the smooth muscle layer in the wall of the uterus.

myopia = nearsightedness, things are seen / focused in the near distance but not in the far distance.

myotome: Gk. mys = muscle, and tome = a cutting; a group of muscles innervated by spinal segment.

myx- mucoid (mix)

Myxoedema AS myxedema (MIX-se-deem-uh) - swelling under the skin due to hypothyroidism - hard oedema (mucoid) in the subcutaneous tissues.

A B C D E F G H I J K L **M** N O P Q R S T U V W X Y Z

A B C D E F G H I J K L M **N** O P Q R S T U V W X Y Z

N

Naevus AS Nevus (NEE-vus) Lt. birthmark, mole circumscribed hyperpigmented tumor of the skin may be pre-cancerous particularly if darkly pigmented.

Nail a thin, hard plate of mostly keratin, derived from the epidermis and develops at the distal end of the fingers and toes.

narc- stupor

nares: plural, Lt. naris = nostril.

nas- nose (nays-)

naris- nose (na-ris-)

naris: Lt. = nostril, plural - nares.

nasal: adj. Lt. nasus = nose; hence, pertaining to the nose.

natal: adj. Lt. natus = born; hence, pertaining of birth.

navicular: Lt. navicula = a little ship; the tarsal bone is concave posteriorly, resembling a boat.

necro- death

Necrosis (neh-KROH-sihs) death of a cell, a group of cells, or a tissue due to disease.

neo-: Gk. prefix - neos = new.

neonatal: adj.Gk. neos = new, & Lt. natos = born; hence, new born

neopallium: Gk. neos = new, and Lt. pallium = cloak; hence, the cerebral cortex which developed more recently than the archipallium or olfactory cortex.

Neoplasm (NEE-OH-plasm) any abnormal growth of tissue or proliferation of cells not under physiological control – may be benign or malignant.

nephro- renal kidney

Nephron (NEH-frohn) the smallest functioning unit of the kidney each of which filters, re-asborbs and secretes the non-protein fluid of the blood.

Nerve an organ of the NS composed of a bundle of neurons, axons and dendrites invested & surrounded by CT and BVs, which functions in the conduction of an impulse from one area of the body to another.

nerve: Lt. nervus = tendon; now a peripheral fibre bundle which conducts impulses to/from the CNS.

Nerve bundle also known as a nerve fasciculus, it is a cord of individual myelinated axons surrounded by perineurium. Numerous bundles compose a single nerve.

Nerve impulse a wave of negative charges (depolarization) that propagates along the outer surface of the plasma membrane of a conductive cell, such as a neuron. (also = an action potential).

Nervous tissue a tissue that consists of two generalized cell types, neurons and neuroglia. Neurons are specialized to initiate action potentials and conduct them at high speeds. Neuroglia provide numerous supportive functions, they are the CT cells of the CNS.

Nerve trunk a combination of nerves that are secured together by epineurium to form a thickened cord of NT.

neur- nerve

neural: adj.Gk. neuron = nerve adj. neurium.

Neurilemma (noo'-rih-LEHM-ah) the outer layer of a myelin sheath associated with a nerve fibre that contains the nucleus and much of the cytoplasm of a Schwann cell.

Neurocranium (new-ROH-kray-NEE-uhm) the part of the skull which houses the brain.

Neuroglia (new'-ROHG-lee-ah) supportive cells of the NS that are most prevalent in the brain and spinal cord. (sing. = pl.)

neuroglia: Gk. neuron = nerve, and glia = glue; the CT of the CNS adj.- neuroglial.

Neurohypophysis: also = the posterior lobe of the pituitary gland. It is composed of NT and is connected to the hypothalamus of the brain by the narrow stalk, the infundibulum. The neurohypophysis receives two hormones released by neurons in the hypothalamus, oxytocin and antidiuretic hormone (ADH).

neurohypophysis: or posterior lobe of hypophysis - Gk. hypo = down, and physis = growth; hence, the posterior part of the hypophysis evaginated downwards from the diencephalon, & its stalk

neurolemma: Gk. neuron = nerve, and lemma = peel or rind; hence, the covering layer of a nerve.

Neuromuscular junction (new'-ro-MUHS-kyoo-lawr JUHNK-shuhn) the area of contact b/n the terminal end of a motor neuron and the sarcolemma of a skeletal muscle fibre.

Neuron (NEW-ron) a cell of NT characterized by its specialization to conduct impulses (conductivity).

neuron: Gk. = nerve; refers to the nerve cell body, with its axon & dendrites; adj- neuronal.

Neurosecretory (new'-roh-seh-KREE-tor-ee) **cells** Neurons that extend from the hypothalamus to the posterior lobe of the pituitary gland and secrete the hormones oxytocin (OT) and antidiuretic hormone (ADH).

Neurotransmitter (new'-ro-TRANS-miht-ah) a molecule that transmits or inhibits the transmission of a nerve impulse from one neuron to another across a synapse.

neutro- neutral

Neutrophil (NEW-tro-fihl) a type of granular, phagocytic WBC characterized by a cytoplasm that stains pink/purple in a neutral stain i.e. does not preferentially take up either acid or base of the stain.

nigra: Lt. niger = black, dark.

noci- pain (noh-see)

node: Lt. nodus = knot.

Node of Ranvier (rahn'-vee-A) a gap in the myelin sheath covering a nerve fibre. It accelerates the rate of impulse conduction.

nodule: diminutive of Lt. nodus = knot, hence, a little knot.

norma: Lt. = pattern or rule, or aspect; adj. normal - according to rule

notch: an indentation in the margin of a structure in organs (e.g. liver, frontal bone).

notochord: Gk. notos = back, and chorde = cord; hence, the primitive axial skeleton around which the vertebrae develop, parts persisting in the nuclei pulposi.

nucha- nape of the neck (new-kah-)

nucha: French nuque = nape or back of the neck; adj.- nuchal.

Nucleolus (new-KLEE-o-luhs) a spherical body w/n the nucleus of a cell, not bound by a plasma membrane. It functions in the storage of ribosomal RNA.

Nucleus (NOO-klee-uhs) the largest structure in a cell. It contains the genetic material to determine protein structure and function, the DNA, and is enveloped by a double-layered plasma membrane. (Also, the dense core of an atom containing protons and neutrons).

nucleus: Lt. = kernel or nut; may refer to the vital centre of a cell body, or to a cluster of neuron cells in the CNS; adj.- nuclear.

nummular Lt nummularis coinlike.

nystagmus: Gk. = drowsiness, to nod, hence, involuntary, rapid, rhythmic eye movements.

O

ob- against, in front of

obex: Lt. = barrier; hence, the coronal fold of ependyma over the lower angle of the 4th ventricle.

Oblique (OH-bleek) slanting or deviated

oblique: adj.Lt. obliquus;= slanting, or deviating from the perpendicular or the horizontal.

oblongata: Lt. oblongus = oblong; medulla oblongata.

obturator: Lt. obturatus = stopped up; hence, a structure which closes a hole.

oc- against, in front of

occiput: Lt. ob = prominent and caput = head; the prominent convexity of the back of the head;

occlusion: Lt. occlusum = closed up; apposition of reciprocal teeth; blocking of any tubular structure;

oculomotor: Lt. oculus = eye, and movere = to move, hence, pertaining to moving the eye.

ocul- eye (ok-ewl)

oculus: Lt. = eye.

oedem- swelling (AS edem-)

odontoid: Gk. odous = tooth, and eidos = form, shape, hence, tooth-like.

oesophagus: Gk. = gullet (passage from pharynx to stomach); adj.- oesophageal.

-oid like

Olecranon (OH-lek-ran-on) to do with the elbow

olecranon: Gk. olene = ulna, and kranion = upper part of head; the upper end of the ulna.

olfactory: adj. Lt. olfacto = smell.

olig- scant, deficent, few, little

olive: Lt. oliva - the oval fruit of the olive tree; oval eminence on medulla oblongata; adj - olivary.

-ology study of

-oma tumor or lump

om(o)- shoulder

om- shoulder

omentum: Lt. = apron; adj.- omental.

omohyoid: Gk. omos = shoulder; hence, a muscle attached to the scapula and hyoid.

onc- cancer

Oncogene (OHN-ko-jeen) a gene that can transform the cell into an oocyte.

Ontogeny (ONn-toj-en-ee) development of an individual growth pattern

onycho- to do with finger and toenails (on-ee-koh)

Oocyte (O-ah-site) A gamete produced within an ovary. (also = ovum or egg).

operculum: Lt. = lid or cover; operculum insulae, the cerebral cortex covering & hiding the insula.

ophthalmic: adj.Gk. ophthalmos = eye.

opponens: Lt. = placing against, opposing.

oppose: Lt. oppositum = put against; hence, to resist or place in contact with.

optic: adj. Gk. optos = seen; hence, pertaining to sight.

Optic disk the area on the retina where the optic nerve exits the eye and contains no rod or cone cells. (also = the blind spot).

or- ora- mouth

ora: Lt. ora = margin or edge.

ora serrata: Lt. ora = margin, and serra = saw; the serrated anterior edge of the retina.

oral: Lt. oris = a mouth, hence, pertaining to the mouth.

orbit: Lt. orbis = circle; the name given to the bony socket in which the eyeball rotates; adj - orbital.

Organ (OR-gan) an organized combination of two or more different types of tissues which performs a general function.

Organ of Corti (KOR-ti) the structure within the inner ear that contains receptor cells sensitive to sound vibrations.

Organelle (or-gan-EHL) a component of a cell that has a consistent, similar structure in other cells and performs a particular function.

Organization - process of wound healing involving the moving in of fibroblasts to pull component parts together

orifice: Lt. orificium = opening.

ortho- straight, straightening (or-thoh)

ortho Gk. orthos = straight combining form meaning straight,

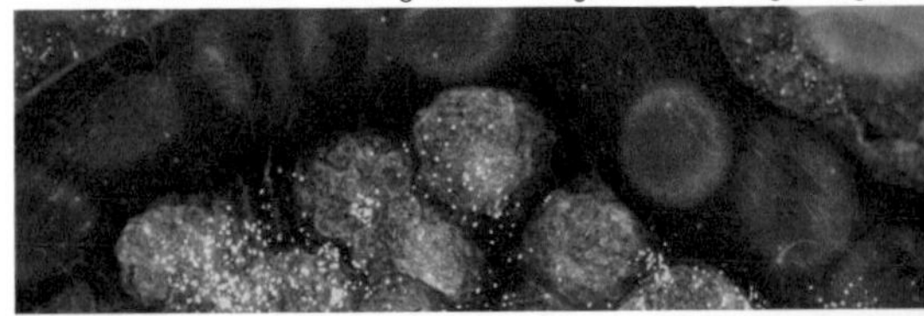

normal, correct
os, oris: Lt. os = mouth; pl. - ora, adj. - oral.
os, ossis: Lt. os = bone; pl. - ossa, adj. - osseous.

-osis condition of / disease of – non-inflammatory

Osseous (OS-ee-uhs) pertaining to bone.
ossicle: Lt. ossiculus, diminutive of os = bone.
ossify: Lt. os = bone, and facio = make; to form bone; and ossification, the process of forming bone

Osteoblast (OS-tee-o-blahst') a type of bone cell characterized by its mobility, its ability to divide and to produce bone matrix.

Osteoclast (OS-tee-o-klahst') a type of bone cell characterized by its ability to dissolve bone matrix.

Osteocyte (OS-tee-o-site') a type of bone cell characterized by its immobile location within a lacunus and by a reduced ability to produce bone matrix.
osteology: Gk. osteon = bone, logy = a field of study.

Osteon (OS-tee-on) an organized arrangement of bone tissue in adult compact bone such that the bone matrix concentrically surrounds a central canal containing a BV. (also = an Haversian system).

Osteonic canal the central canal in an osteon that contains a BV. (also = Haversian canal).

-osteum pertaining to bone (os-tee-um)
osteum: Lt. pertaining to bone.
ostium: Lt. = a door, an opening, an orifice.

ot- ear
otic: adj.Gk. otos = ear.

Otoliths small calcium carbonate crystals located w/n the maculae of the inner ear's utricle and saccule. The otoliths move in response to head movements, shifting their mass which distorts the hair cell processes. As a result, nerve impulses are generated to the brain for interpretation as head movements for static equilibrium.
otolith: Gk. otos = ear, and lithos = stone; hence, calcareous particles in the utricle and saccule of the membranous labyrinth.

Ovary (OH-vahr-ee) the female gonad, or primary reproductive organ that produces gametes and female sex hormones
ovary: Lt. ovum = egg; hence, the organ containing ova (the largest cells in the female).
ovum: Lt. = egg, plural - ova.

oxy- sharp

A B C D E F G H I J K L M N O P Q R S T U V W X Y Z

P

Pacinian corpuscle (pa-SIHN-ee-an KOR-puhs-ehl) a receptor located in the dermis that responds to touch (pressure).

pachy- thick (pak-ee)

paed- child

palate: Lt. palatum = palate, adj.- palatal.

paleo: Gk. palaios = old; hence, paleocerebellum, the earliest stage in the evolution of the cerebellum.

pali- recurrence

pallidus: adj.Lt. = pale.

pallium: Lt. = cloak:, the cerebral cortex forming the outer covering of the cerebral hemisphere.

palma: Lt. palma = palm; adj, palmar - Lt. palmaris.

palpate: Lt. palpare = to touch, and palpatus = touched; to examine by feeling, and palpation.

palpebra: Lt. = eyelid,

pampiniform: adj. Lt. pampinus = tendril, and forma = shape.

pan- general overall

Pancreas (PAN-kree-as) a soft, oblong organ located posterior to the stomach in the abdominal cavity. The pancreas secretes digestive enzymes and hormones that regulate blood sugar.

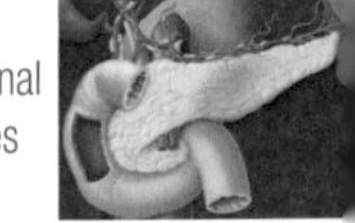

pancreas: Gk. = sweetbread, derived from Gk. pan = all, and kreas = flesh; adj. pancreatic.

panniculus: diminutive of Lt. pannus = cloth.

Papilla (paw-PIHL-ah) a small finger-shaped projection.

papilla: Lt. = nipple or teat; adj.- papillary.

par- beside

para- against, aside, abnormal, unequal

paradidymis: Gk. para = beside of near, & didymis = twinned or paired, refers to testes; the collection of convoluted tubules in the spermatic cord, above the head of the epididymis.

paraesthesia: Gk. para = beside, and aisthesia = sensation; abnormal sensation, eg burning or pricking.

paralysis: Gk. para = beside, near, lyein = to loosen; loss or impairment of muscle function.

parametrium: Gk. para = beside, & metra = womb; CT within the broad ligament alongside the uterus.

paraplegia: Gk. para = beside, and plege = a stroke; paralysis c the lower limbs.

pararenal: adj. Gk para = beside, Lt. ren = kidney; beside the kidney, eg, pararenal fat, the fatty capsule of the kidney

Parasagittal (pahr'-ah-SAHJ-ih-tahl) A plane that extends vertically through the body dividing it into unequal right and left portions.

parasternal: adj. Gk. para = beside, and sternon = chest; the parasternal line is a vertical line midway b/n the sternal edge & the midclavicular line.

Parasympathetic division (pahr'-ah-sihmp-ah-THEH-tihk dih-VISH-zhuhn) the component of the ANS that stimulates activities which conserve body energy and direct BF to the GIT &/or the sexual organs. The nerves synapse "beside" the organs they affect.

Paralysis - total or partial loss of movement due to interruption of the nerve signal - often a partial paralysis is referred to as a palsy or paresis, which are corruptions of the term.

parasympathetic: adj. Gk para = beside, syn = with, & pathos = feeling; part of the autonomic NS which is complementary to the sympathetic NS

Parathyroid (pahr'-ah-THI-royd) **gland** One of 4 or 5 pea-shaped glands located embedded into the posterior side of the thyroid gland.

parathyroid: adj. Gk. para = beside, (thyroid); beside the thyroid gland.

Parenchyma (par'-EN-kihm-ah) the functioning elements of an organ as opposed to the structural or supporting elements (also ≠ stroma)

parenchyma: Gk. para = beside or near, en = in, and chein = to pour; designating the functional elements of an organ, as opposed to the framework or stroma.

paresis: Gk. = relaxation, but has come to mean partial paralysis.

Parietal (pa-RI-eh-tal) pertaining to the outer wall of a cavity or organ e.i. parietal layer of the pericardium, outer of the 2 layers of the pericardium ≠ visceral.

parietal: adj. Lt. parietalis, pertaining to paries = wall.

Parietal cell a cell in the stomach mucosa that secretes hydrochloric acid and intrinsic factor.

Parietal pericardium (peh-ree-KARD-ee-um) the outer serous membrane covering the heart. (also = the pericardial sac).

Parietal pleura (PLEW-rah) the outer serous membrane associated with each lung. It is attached to the inner thoracic wall.

Paronychia (Pa-ron-IK-ee-uh) a bacterial infection of the skin near the nail.

Parotid (pah-ROHT-ihd) **glands** a pair of salivary glands, each of

A B C D E F G H I J K L M N O **P** Q R S T U V W X Y Z

which is located between the skin of the cheek and the masseter muscle on a side of the face.

parotid: adj. Gk. para = beside, and otos = of the ear; hence, beside the ear.

parous: adj. Lt. pario = I bear (children); adj. applied to women who have borne children ≠ nulliparous,

pars: Lt. = part.

part- childbirth

patella: Lt. a small pan; adj.- patellar.

path-/ -pathy disease / disease of

Pathogenesis- origin or cause of a diseae.

path- disease, Pathology (pahth-OH-loh-jee) the study or science of diseases.

Pathology (pahth-OH-loh-jee) the study or science of diseases.

pecten: Lt. = comb.

pectinate: adj. from Lt. pecten = a comb; applied to structures having the appearance of parallel teeth arising from a straight back (eg. musculi pectinati) pectineal: adj.

pectineus: Lt., pecten = a comb; hence the muscle attaching to the pecten (pectineal line) of the pubic bone.

pectoral: adj. Lt. pectoris = of the front of the chest.

pectoralis: adj. Lt. pectoris = of the front of the chest.

pedicle: diminutive of Lt. pedis = of the foot.

pedis: Lt. = of the foot.

peduncle: variation of pedicle.

Pellagra (PEL-lag-ruh) Lt, pelle = skin, agros = rough - rough skin. description of skin roughened by lack of niacin=nicotinic acid.

pellucidum: adj. Lt. per = through, & lucere - to shine; translucent.

pelvis: Lt. = basin, adj.- pelvic.

pemphigus : Gk. pemphix = blister (PEM-fix)

Penis (PEE-nihs) the external reproductive organ of the male through which most of the urethra extends.

-penia lack of

penis: Lt. = tail, the male organ of copulation (cf. appendix, appendage).

pennate: Lt. penna = feather; hence, a muscle whose fibres approach the tendon from one direction is unipennate; from two, bipennate, and from more than two, multipennate.

pennatus: (pinnate) - adj. Lt. penna = feather; hence, a muscle whose fibres approach the tendon from one direction is unipennate; from two, bipennate, and from >2, multipennate.

per- through / excessive

peri- around, about / beyond

perianal: adj.Gk. peri = around, and Lt. anus = lower opening of alimentary canal.

Pericardial (pear'-ih-KAR-dee-ahl) **cavity** a narrow space b/n the outer wall of the heart (the visceral pericardium) & the parietal pericardium. It contains pericardial fluid.

Pericardium (pear'-ih-KAR-dee-uhm) the serous membrane associated with the heart, composed of two layers, an inner visceral pericardium and an outer parietal pericardium.

pericardium: Gk. peri = around, and kardia = heart; hence, the membranes enclosing the heart.

Perichondrium (pear'-ih-KOHN-dree-uhm) a layer of dense CT that envelopes cartilage.

perichondrium: Gk. peri = around, and chondros = cartilage; hence, the membrane covering cartilage.

pericranium: Gk. peri = around, and kranion = skull; hence, the external periosteum of the skull.

perilymph: Gk. peri = around, & lympha - Lt. = clear water; the fluid in the bony labyrinth surrounding the membranous labyrinth (and continuous with the CSF).

Perimysium (pear'-ih-MI-see-uhm) an extension of the epimysium of muscle that invaginates inward to divide a muscle into bundles.

perineum: Gk. the caudal aspect of the trunk b/n the thighs, or, the region of the trunk below the pelvis

Perineurium (pear'-ih-NYEW-ree-uhm) an extension of the epineurium of a nerve that invaginates inward to wrap around bundles of nerve fibres.

pelvic diaphragm; adj.- perineal.

periodontal: adj.Gk. peri = around, and odont = tooth.

Periodontal ligament (pear'-ee-o-DON-tal LIG-ah-ment) a CT membrane that surrounds a tooth and connects it to the bone of the jaw

Periosteum (pear'-ee-OS-tee-uhm) the CT covering around a bone that is important in bone growth, nutrition, and repair.

periosteum: Gk. peri = around, and osteon = bone; the membrane around a bone.

Peripheral (per-IH-fehr-ahl) **nervous system** (**PNS**) The division of the NS consisting of nerves and ganglia located between the CNS and the body surfaces.

A B C D E F G H I J K L M N O **P** Q R S T U V W X Y Z

A B C D E F G H I J K L M N O **P** Q R S T U V W X Y Z

peripheral: adj.Gk. peri = around and phero = carry; away from the centre (c.f. periphery).

peristalsis: Gk. peri = around, & stellein - to constrict; a circular constriction passing as a wave along a muscular tube; adj.- peristaltic.

Peritoneal (pear'-ih-to-NEE-awl) **cavity** the space between the parietal peritoneum and the visceral peritoneum. It contains a small amount of fluid.

Peritoneum (per'-ih-to-NEE-uhm) the extensive serous membrane associated with the abdominopelvic cavity.

peritoneum: Gk. periteino = to stretch around; the membrane stretched around the internal surface of the walls & the external aspect of some of the contents of the abdomen; adj.- peritoneal.

pero- stunted, malformed

Peroxisomes (pehr-OHX-ih-sohmz) small, spherical cellular organelles similar to lysosomes that play catabolic roles in the cell.

peroneal: adj.Gk. perone = clasp, brooch - see fibula.

pes: Lt. = foot.

petr- rock, stone

petrosal: adj.Lt. petrosus = rocky. / petrous: adj.Lt. petrosus = rocky.

Peyer's patches (PA-yehrz PAH-chuhz) clusters of lymphatic tissue (farj-) containing numerous WBC that are located in the wall of the small intestine.

phaeo- dusky AS pheo- (FAY-oh)

phag- eater

Phagocyte (FAY-go-cite) Gk phago- = to eat kyte = cell which ingests matter.

Phagocytosis (fayg'-o-sih-TO-sihs) a type of cytosis in which bulk solid materials may be transported into a cell. It is performed by WBCs for the removal of harmful particles and cells from the body. Large groups of WBCs may coalese to form Giant cells to engulf large particles such as cotton fibres.

phalang- fingers or toes (falanj-)

phalanx: Lt. = row of soldiers; one of the small bones of a digit, pl- phalanges, adj.- phalangeal.

phallus: Gk. phallos = penis.

phan- appear visible

phao- brown, dusky(FAY-oh)

Pharynx (FAHR-ihnks) a tube that extends from the level of the internal nares to its union with the larynx, which transports air, food, & liquid.

pharynx: Gk. = throat; adj.- pharyngeal.

phas- appear visible, speak, utter (FAZ)

phen- light, bright, manifest

-phil love of

philtrum: Gk. philtron - the median sulcus of the upper lip.

phleb- vein (FLEB)

Phlegm (FLEM) = (sputum) mucous arising from the lungs - thought to originally come from BVs.

-phobe hate of

phleg- inflammation

phon- voice

phonation: Gk. phone = sound or voice; the production of either.

photo- light (FOH-toh) (replaced now by radio- in imaging).

phren- mind, diaphragm

phrenic: Gk. phren = diaphragm or mind; hence, diaphragmatic (cf. schizophrenic).

physi- natural (fizz-ee)

pia: Lt. = faithful, the membrane which faithfully follows the contour of the brain and SC. = soft

Pia mater (PE-ah MA-tehr) The innermost of the three meninges surrounding the brain and SC.

pilomotor: Lt. pilus = a hair, & movere = to move; the action of the arrectores pilorum muscles.

pilus: Lt. = a hair adj pilar see also tricho.

Pineal (pie-NEE-ahl) **gland** a small endocrine gland located at the posterior end of the diencephalon, forming a part of the roof of the third ventricle. (also = the epithalamus).

pineal: adj. Lt. pinea = a pine cone; hence, the pineal gland which is cone-shaped.

Pinocytosis (pihn'-o-sih-TO-sihs) a type of exocytosis in which bulk amounts of fluid are transported into the cell.

piriform: adj. Lt. pirum = a pear; hence, pear-shaped.

pisiform: adj. Lt. pisum = a pea; hence, pea-shaped.

pityriasis: n Gk. pityrus = bran hence, bran flake generally on the skin (PIT-ee-rye-a-sis)

pituitary: Lt. pituita = mucous or phlegm, the gland was thought to produce mucous which was discharged through the nose.

Pituitary (pih-TEW-ih-tahr-ee) **gland** a small, functionally important endocrine gland located inferior to the hypothalamus and attached to it by way of a short stalk. (also = the hypophysis).

placenta: Lt. = a flat, round cake.

placode: Gk. plax = plate or flat, and eidos = shape or form.

plan- flat, level, to wander

-plasia growth

Plasma (PLAZ-mah) - fluid formed when blood settles w/o clotting - clotting factors present- (as opposed to serum when the blood clots and the remaining fluid is serum - clotting factors all used up.)

plane: Lt. planus = flat; hence, a real or imaginary flat surface.

planta: Lt. the sole of the foot; adj.- plantar or plantaris.

plantar: adj. Lt. planta = the sole of the foot.

Plasma (PLAHZ-mah) the extracellular fluid that forms a portion of blood.

Plasma membrane a microscopic barrier associated with cells composed mainly of a phospholipid bilayer and protein. The outer plasma membrane of a cell is also called the cell membrane.

plat- broad, flat

Platelet (PLA-teh-leht) a formed element of blood that is active in blood clot formation.

platysma: Gk. = flat object; the flat, subcutaneous muscle extending from below the clavicle to the mouth.

pleo- many (plee-oh-)

pleur- lungs, respiratory

Pleura (PLEW-rah) the serous membrane associated with the lungs. It consists of an inner visceral layer and an outer parietal layer.

pleura: Gk. = a rib. Later used to name the serous membrane lining the chest walls and the lungs.

Pleural cavity a narrow space between the visceral and parietal pleurae that contains pleural fluid.

Plexus (PLEHKS-uhs) a network of interconnecting nerves, veins, or lymphatic vessels.

plexus: Lt. = a network or plait.

plica: Lt. plicare = to fold; hence, a fold.

pluri- several

pne-/pneu (new) air, to breathe

pne- air, breathe (new)

pneumon: Gk. pneuma = air.

pod-/podia foot / formation of a foot for movement

Podocyte (PO-doh-site) a fenestrated cell forming the visceral layer of Bowman's capsule in the kidneys.

poikilo- irregular

A B C D E F G H I J K L M N O **P** Q R S T U V W X Y Z

polio- grey (poh-lih-oh)

pollex- thumb

pollex: Lt. = thumb.

pollicis: genitive (possessive case) of Lt. pollex = thumb; hence of the thumb.

poly- many

Polyp (PO-lip) structure with stalk and rounded, swollen head

pompholyx Gk = bubble used to describe a blistering on the skin (POM-fo-lix)

Pons (pohnz) a part of the brain located between the midbrain and the medulla oblongata.

pons: Lt. = bridge; adj.- pontine; part of the brain stem.

pont- bridge

popliteus: Lt. poples = the ham or thigh, and sometimes, the knee; adj.popliteal, referring to the fossa behind the knee or its contents.

por- passageway

porta: Lt. = a gate, also Lt. portare = to carry; hence, the portal system carries venous blood from the alimentary tract to the porta hepatis; adj.- portal.

porus: Lt. a pore or foramen; hence, the openings of the acoustic meatuses.

post- after, behind

postero- posterior part

Posterior (po-STEER-ee-or) a directional term describing the location of a part being toward the back or rear side relative to another part. In humans it is also known as dorsal.

posterior: adj. Lt. post = behind (in place or time).

Posterior horn a region of the SC grey matter containing sensory neuron cell bodies. (also = the ventral horn).

Posterior root the structure merging with the SC on its posterior aspect that contains sensory nerves. (also = the dorsal root).

Posterior pituitary gland the part of the pituitary gland at the base of the brain consisting of the axons of neurons originating in the hypothalamus and supporting tissue.

posture: Lt. positus = placed; hence, the position of the body as a whole at a given moment, e.g. erect, recumbent, prone, supine, sitting, kneeling.

prae- in front of, before

pre- in front of, before

precuneus: Lt. pre = before, and cuneus = wedge; the parietal lobule anterior to the cuneus.

prepuce: Lt. praeputium = foreskin (of penis or clitoris).

presby- old

prim- first

Primary germ layer One of 3 layers of cells that differentiate during the embryonic stage to give rise to all tissues in the body. They are the endoderm, mesoderm, and ectoderm.

princeps: Lt. primus = chief, & capere = to take; hence chief or principal.

procerus: Lt. = slender, elongated; hence, the vertical slip of muscle between the medial part of frontalis & the root of the nose.

pro- in front of

Process (PROH-sehs) general term used to describe any marked projection or prominence.

process/processus: Lt. = going forwards, indicating growing out, ie. an outgrowth, usually bone e.g., the zygomatic process of the temporal.

proct- anus, rectum

profundus: Lt. pro = before, and fundus = bottom; hence profundus = deep.

Prognosis (prog-NOH-sis) the expected outcome of a disease.

prognosis Gk. pro= in front of gno= to know – fore knowledge.

prominens: Lt. = projecting.

promontory: Lt. promontorium = a headland, ie. part of land jutting into the sea - a bony prominence.

pronate: Lt. pronatus = bent forwards; to pronate = to turn the hand so that the palm faces downwards or posteriorly supinate.

prone: Lt. pronatus = bent forwards; recumbent face-down posture.

pronus- face down

proprioceptive: Lt. proprius = one's own, and captum = taken; sensory impulses received by the joints and muscles within one's own body.

pros- forward, anterior

prosection: Lt. pro = before, and sectum = cut. A dissection to demonstrate anatomic structures.

prosector: Lt. pro = before, and sectum = cut. One who prepares an anatomical dissection.

prosencephalon: Lt. pro = in front, and Gk. enkephalos = brain; part of the brain rostral to the midbrain.

Prostate (PROH-stat) **gland** a walnut-shaped gland surrounding the urethra as it emerges from the urinary bladder in males. Its secretions contribute to semen.

prostate: Gk. pro = before, & Lt. = statum = stood; something which stands before - e.g. the prostate gland stands before the urinary bladder.

protract: Lt. protractus = drawn out; hence, to put forwards (e.g., shoulder or mandible). Protraction - the act of protracting.

protrude: Lt. protrudo = thrust forwards, e.g. the tongue; protrusion - the act of protruding.

protuberance: Lt. protubero = I bulge out; hence, a bulging bony feature (see tuber).

Proximal (PROHKS-ih-mal) a directional term indicating a body part that is located nearer to the origin or point of attachment to the trunk than another; opposite of distal.

proximal: adj. Lt. proxime = nearest; hence, nearer to the root of a limb.

pseudo- false (syoo-doh)

Pseudopod (SOO-do-pohd) a streaming extension of plasma membrane-bound cytoplasm from a mobile cell.

Pseudostratified (sew'-do-STRAHT-ih-fide) pertaining to a single layer of epithelial cells which appears multi-layered when viewed in a prepared slide.

pseudostratified Lt. pseudo = false stratified = multi-layered.

psor- itching (saw-)

psoas: Gk. = loin.

Psoriasis (SAW-rye-uh-sis) a spongiform chronic irritating dermatitis occurring on the extensor surfaces of the skin.

pter- wing (ter-)

pterion: Gk. pteron = wing; the region where the tip of the greater wing of the sphenoid meets or is close to the parietal, separating the frontal from the squamous temporal; alternatively the region where these 4 bones meet.

Pterygium (TER-rij-ee-um) triangular fleshy mass of thickened conjunctiva growing in the inner aspect of the eyeball – may grow over the cornea and affect the vision.

pterygoid: adj.Gk. pteryx = wing, and eidos = shape; hence, wing-shaped.

ptosis: Gk. = fall; hence, drooping of an eyelid, or descent of an internal organ.

puberty: Lt. puber = adult; hence, the time when hair appears in the pubic region - i.e., near the pubis - as a secondary sexual characteristic.

pubes: Lt. = adult or signs of manhood, hence the lower

abdominal secondary sexual hair.

pudendal: adj.Lt. pudendus = shameful; hence, pertaining to the external genitalia.

pulmonary: adj.Lt. pulmo = lung.

pulp: Lt. pulpa = a soft part of the body or tooth.

Pulp cavity the space w/n a tooth that is filled with pulp, which consists of CT containing BVs & Ns.

pulposus: Lt. pulpa = a soft part of the body or tooth, hence pulpy or soft.

pulvinar: Lt. pulvinus = rounded cushion; the posterior end of the thalamus.

punctum: Lt. = a sharp point; hence a very small point or orifice.

pupil: Lt. pupilla = the central black orifice in the iris; adj.- pupillary.

Pupil (PYOO-pihl) the small hole through the centre of the iris in the eye through which light passes.

Purkinje cells Large, highly branched neurons in the cerebellar cortex that receive input from many thousands of synapses.

purpur- purple

Purpura (PURR-purr-uh) a non-blanchable rash where the RBCs are trapped beneath the skin so giving it a purple appearance

Pus (Lt) liquid product of inflammation – with cell fragments particularly inflammatory cells. Pustule diminutive of pus.

putamen: Lt. = peel, husk or shell of fruit or seed (the external part of the lentiform nucleus).

pyelo- basin , pelvis (generally renal pelvis)

pyelogram: Gk. pyelos = basin, and gramma = diagram; hence, radiograph of the renal pelvis (and usually of the ureter) after filling with contrast medium.

Pyemia (PEYE-ee-muh) septicemia with pus in the blood ± sites of suppuration throughout the body.

pykno- thick, dense

pyo- pus

pylorus: Gk. = gate-keeper; hence, the part of the pyloric canal containing the sphincter, which guards the opening into the duodenum; adj.- pyloric.

pyramid: Gk. pyramis = a pyramid (solid with 3- or more-sided base, and flat sides.

Pyramidal cells neurons w/n the cerebral cortex of the brain which initiate somatic motor impulses.

A B C D E F G H I J K L M N O **P** Q R S T U V W X Y Z

Q

quad- four

quadrangular: Lt. quadri = four and angulus = angle; hence square or rectangular.
quadratus: Lt. = square or rectangular.
quadriceps: Lt. quadri = four, and caput = head; hence, a 4-headed muscle.
quadrigeminus: Lt. quadri = four, & gemini = paired or twinned; hence four-fold.

R

rachi- spine, vertebral column

Rash any change in the skin which affects appearance, colour or texture.

radi- root, spine, radiation

radiation: Lt. radiatus = radiant; hence, divergence from a common centre (c.f. radius).

radicle: diminutive of Lt. radix = root; hence a small root, adj.- radicular.

radius: Lt. = spoke of a wheel, which rotates around the hub; hence, the lateral bone of the forearm, which rotates (though around an almost vertical axis); adj.- radial.

radix: Lt. = root.

ramify: Lt. ramus = a branch; & facere = to make; hence, to branch

rami- branch (ray-mee)

ramus: Lt. = branch; hence, a branch of a nerve, bone or blood vessel.

raphe: Gk. a seam; hence, the line of junction of the edges of 2 muscles or areas of skin.

re- return, back again

Receptor (ree-SEHP-tor) a structure that is capable of responding to a stimulus by initiating a nerve impulse.

recess: Lt. recessus = a secluded area or pocket;a small cavity set apart from a main cavity.

rectum: adj.Lt. rectus = straight. (The rectum was named in animals where it is straight - not so in Man).

rectus: Lt. rectus = straight.

recurrent: Lt. re = back, and currere = to run; hence a structure which bends, then runs back to its source.

Red bone marrow a CT located within spongy bone which contains the stem cells & their differentiated forms involved in blood cell formation.

Red pulp: part of the interior areas of the spleen (the other is white pulp). Red pulp serves as a storage area for erythrocytes (RBCs), and consists of venous sinuses and cords of CT known as splenic cords. This is contractile in rodents and allows for the release of blood in shock conditions.

reflex: an involuntary response - muscular or secretory - to a stimulus mediated by the CNS.

Region (REE-jon) an area often of the abdomen defined by anatomical surface markers, used to enter the abdomen or to locate pain or an abnormality smaller than a zone or zona.

ren- kidney

Renal (REE-nawl) pertaining to the kidneys.

renal: adj.Lt. ren = kidney.

Renal corpuscle (REE-nal KOR-puhs-ehl) the portion of a kidney nephron consisting of the Bowman's capsule and glomerulus. (see Corpuscle).

Renal cortex the outer part of a kidney, which contains renal corpuscles and segments of renal tubules.

Renal medulla the inner part of a kidney. It contains renal tubules and BVs. W/n the renal medulla are the renal pyramids, which are striated pyramid-shaped areas formed by the congregation of renal tubules

Renal pelvis (REE-nal PEHL-vihs) a membrane-lined basin w/n the renal sinus of each kidney.

Renal pyramid (REE-nal PEER-a-mihd) One of about 8 to 10 cone-shaped structures in each kidney extending from the medulla to the cortex, which contain the renal tubules.

Renal sinus (REE-nal SI-nuhs) a potential space w/n each kidney extending from the hilum to the medulla. It contains the renal pelvis.

Renal tubule (REE-nal TEW-byewl) part of a nephron of the kidney consisting of a simple epithelial lined tube extending from Bowman's capsule to a collecting duct. There are 3 parts to each tubule: the proximal convoluted tubule, the Loop of Henle (= renal loop) and the distal convoluted tubule. The functions of reabsorption, secretion, concentration or dilution occur across the walls.

Respiratory membrane the barrier in the lungs which must be crossed by gas molecules during gas exchange. It consists of the alveolar epithelium, a BM, and the endothelium of a capillary.

rete: Lt. = a net; hence, a network of veins or tubules.

reticular: adj.Lt. reticulum = small net; hence having a network.

reticulum: diminutive of Lt. rete = net; adj.- reticular.

Retina (REHT-ih-nah) the light-sensitive inner layer of the eye containing rod and cone cells.

retina: derivation uncertain - the innermost of the 3 layers of the eyeball.

retinaculum: Lt. = a tether; hence, a thickened band of deep fascia which retains tendons or the patella.

retract: Lt. re = back, and tractum = pulled; to pull something back, and retraction - the act of retracting.

A B C D E F G H I J K L M N O P Q **R** S T U V W X Y Z

retro- located behind

retro: prefix - Lt. = backwards.

retroflexion: Lt. retro = backwards, and flexion = bent; the position of being bent backwards, applied to the angulation of the body of the uterus on the cervix.

retroversion: Lt. retro = backwards, and version = turned; the position of being turned backwards, applied to the angulation of the cervix uteri on the vagina.

rhabdo- striated, striped

rhe- flow

rheum- mucoid or watery discharge / relating to joint pain

rhin- nose

rhinencephalon: Gk. rhinion = nostril, & enkephalos = brain; the brain tissue concerned with smell.

rhombencephalon: Gk. rhombos = rhomboid, & enkephalos = brain; hence, the hind-brain: consisting of the medulla oblongata, pons and cerebellum, which enclose the rhomboid fossa (floor of 4th ventricle).

rhod- red

rhomboid: adj. Gk. rhombus = a figure with 4 equal sides, not at right angles, the shape of a rhombus.

Ribosome (RYE-boh-zome) a microscopic, spherical structure w/n the cytoplasm of a cell composed of RNA and protein. It serves as an attachment site for messenger RNA during protein synthesis.

Ridge (RID-je) elevated growth often roughened.

rigor- Lt. rigor = stiffness

rima: Lt. = chink; hence, e.g., rima palpebrarum = the chink b/n the free edges of the eyelids.

risorius: Lt. risor = scoffer; risorius is the "smiling" muscle drawing the corners of the mouth laterally.

Rod cell a photoreceptor cell in the retina of the eye that detects very low levels of light.

rostral: adj. Lt. rostrum = beak, implying nearness to the corpus callosum.

rostrum: Lt. beak, a platform or beak-like structure; adj.- rostral.

rotate: Lt. rota = wheel; hence, to turn, and rotation, the act of turning.

rotundum: Lt. rotnudus = round.

rub- red

rubro: prefix, Lt. rubrum = red.

ruga: Lt. = a wrinkle.

rugose: adj. Lt. ruga = a wrinkle, hence, wrinkled.

S

sac: Lt. saccus = a sack.
saccule: Lt. sacculus, diminutive of saccus.
sacrum: Lt. sacer = sacred (probably considered so because of its size).

Sagittal (SAJ-ih-tal) a vertical plane that divides the body into right and left portions, & includes the midsagittal/median sagittal plane (dividing into equal halves) and the parasagittal plane (dividing into unequal portions).

sagittal: adj. Lt. sagitta = arrow, because the sagittal suture is notched posteriorly, like an arrow, by the lambdoid sutures.

Salivary (SAHL-ih-vahr-ee) **gland** one of several exocrine glands in the facial region that secrete saliva into the mouth to initiate the digestive process.

salivary: adj. Lt. saliva = spit.

salping- tube

salpinx: Gk. = trumpet; the uterine or auditory tubes, each of which is trumpet-shaped.
saphenous: adj. Gk. saphenes = obviously visible.
The saphenous veins become obvious when varicose.

Sarcolemma (sar'-ko-LEHM-ah) the plasma membrane covering the outer surface of a muscle fibre.

Sarcoma (SAR-coh-mah) Gk sarcoma = fleshy, -oma = tumor, used to describe a malignant tumor derived from connective tissue

Sarcomere (SAR-ko-meer) a contractile microscopic subunit of striated muscle (skeletal and cardiac muscle).

Sarcoplasm (SAHR-ko-plahzm) the cytoplasm of a muscle fibre.

Sarcoplasmic reticulum (sahr'-koh-PLAHZ-mihk reh-TIHK-yew-luhm) a cellular organelle found only in muscle cells that stores calcium ions, and is similar in structure to the endoplasmic reticulum found in other cells. (see also endoplasmic reticulum).

sartorius: Lt. = tailor:, sartorius muscles, when contracted produce the tailor's posture; squatting.
scalene: adj. Gk. skalenos = uneven, hence a triangle with unequal sides, a description of the scalenus anterior and scalenus medius muscles.
scaphoid: adj. Gk. skaphe = skiff, and eidos = shape or form; hence the carpal bone which is hollowed out on its distal surface

for the head of the capitate; also the fossa occupied by tensor veli palatine muscle.

scapula: Gk. skapto = I dig, - because of the resemblance to a spade.

scar (Gk. escara = scab) remnants of healing.

scel- leg

schiz- split

Schwann cell a type of neuroglial cell that forms myelin sheaths around axons of peripheral nerves.

Sciatic (SY-at-ic) nerve, largest nerve in the body lies on the ischium and is very visible hence the name sciatic pain, resulting from damage to the sciatic nerve or parts of it

sciatic: adj.Gk. ischion = hip-joint. Ischiadikos meant pertaining to the ischium or hip - later changed to ischium. (the ischium earns its name because it forms > 2/5 of the acetabulum, whereas the ilium contributes < 2/5, and the pubis only 1/5). The sciatic nerve lies on the ischium.

scirrho- hard

sclero- hard

Sclera (SKLEH-raw) the posterior part of the outer, fibrous tunic covering the eyeball; the white of the eye.

sclera: Gk. skleros = hard; hence the tough, outer layer of the eyeball; adj.- scleral.

scolio- twisted

scoliosis: Gk. skolios = crooked or curved, and -osis = condition, hence, the lateral curvature of the spine.

scrotum: possibly derived from Lt. scorteus = leather; adj. scrotal.

sebum wax, oil

Sebaceous (seh-BAY-shuhs) **gland** an exocrine gland located in the dermis that secretes an oily substance called sebum. It is usually associated with a hair follicle.

second- second following

secrete: Lt. secretus = separated; hence, to produce a chemical substance by glandular activity - adj. -secretory; noun, secretion.

Secretion (seh-KREE-shuhn) a substance produced and released by a cell that serves a useful benefit.

sella: Lt. = saddle; adj.- sellar, sella turcica = Turkish saddle.

semen: Lt. = seed; adj.- seminal (seminal vesicle).

semi- half, partial

semilunaris: adj.Lt. semi = half, and luna = moon; hence, having a half-moon shape.

Semicircular canal (seh'-mi-SEHR-kyoo-lawr caw-NAHL) one of three looping canals in each temporal bone that form a part of the inner ear. It contains perilymph fluid and the receptors for equilibrium.

semimembranosus: adj. Lt. semi = half, and membrana = membrane; hence, the hamstring muscle of which the upper half is membranous.

Seminal vesicle (SEHM-ih-nawl VEHS-ih-kehl) one of a pair of convoluted glands of the male reproductive system located posterior to the urinary bladder that secretes part of the semen.

seminiferous: Lt. semen = seed and ferre = to carry, to bear: the sperm-producing tubules in the testes.

Seminiferous tubule (sehm'-i-NIHF-ehr-uhs TEW-byewl) a microscopic, tightly packed tube w/n each testis where the sperm cells develop.

semitendinosus: adj. Lt. semi = half, and tendo = I stretch; - the hamstring muscle (the lower half is tendinous).

seps- decay

septum: Lt. saeptum = fenced in; hence, a dividing fence or partition - generally of CT.

Serosa (sehr-O-sah) any serous membrane (also, the outer membranous layer of a visceral organ containing blood & nerve supply as well as lymphatic drainage), similar to the capsule of an organ.

serous: Lt. = like serum, serum-like.

Serous membrane (SEHR-uhs MEHM-brane) an epithelial membrane that lines a body cavity or covers an organ, and secretes small amounts of fluid.

serratus: adj. Lt. = notched like the edge of a saw (serrate).

Serum - (SEE-rum) fluid formed when blood clots see plasma.

sesamoid: adj. Gk. sesamodes, eidos = shape or form; like grains of sesame, ie. small bone in tendon at site of friction.

sialogram: Gk. sialon = saliva, and gramma = a diagram; hence, a radiograph of a salivary duct.

sicc- dry

sigmoid: adj. Gk. sigma, the form used at the end of a word having an S-shape; hence, S-shaped.

sinister: adj. Lt. = left-sided.

Sigmoid colon (SIHG-moyd KOH-luhn) the distal segment of the colon located b/n the descending colon & the rectum.

sign - objective evidence of disease / as opposed to symptom - a subjective reporting of disease.

Simple (SIHM-pehl) pertaining to a single-layered arangement of epithelial cells.

Sinoatrial node (sin'-oh-AY-tree-awl nohd) (**SA node**) a cluster of specialized cardiac muscle cells in the wall of the right atrium that initiate each cardiac cycle (also = the sinuatrial node, or pacemaker).

sinistro-left

Sinus (SEYE-nuhs) a space w/n a bone lined with mucous membrane, such as the frontal and maxillary sinuses in the head. (also, a modified BV usually vein with an enlarged lumen for blood storage and containing no or little muscle in its wall).

sinus: Lt. = a hollow or space which may contain air, venous or arterial blood, lymph or serous fluid; adj.sinusoid.

pathologically - suppurating channel or fistula.

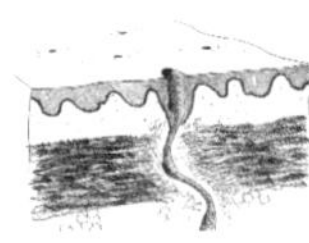

Sinusoids an extensive network of vessels that may be found in the liver, pancreas, spleen, and adrenal cortex, which are similar in structure to capillaries only "leakier".

Skeletal muscle tissue one of 3 types of muscle tissue in the body characterized by the presence of visible organized striations and under conscious control over its contraction. It attaches to bones to form the muscles of the body.

Skull (sk-UHL) this a term for all the bones of the head

Small intestine the organ of the alimentary canal located b/n the stomach and the large intestine that functions in the final digestion, filtration and absorption of nutrients.

Smooth muscle one of 3 types of muscle tissue in the body characterized by the lack of visible striations, with automatic and autonomic contractile function. It forms part of the walls of hollow organs and BVs.

solar Gk sol = sun to do with the sun see also actinic

sole: the lower surface of the foot - see soleus.

soleus: adj. Lt. solea = flatfish or sandal; soleus muscle does not enter the sole of the foot, but resembles the fish.

solitarius: Lt. = solitary, alone.

Soma (SOH-mah) pertaining to the body or the main part of an organ or a cell

soma: Gk. = the body.

somatic: adj.Gk. soma = the body; hence, pertaining to the body frame but not to its viscera.

Somatic nervous system the component of the PNS that conveys impulses associated with conscious sensory and motor activities.

somite: Gk. soma = body, hence an embryonic body segment.

somn- sleep

Sore (SOR) = ulcer skin defect involving all levels.

spano- few, scanty

spasm: Gk. spasmos = an involuntary contraction of a muscle; adj.- spastic, or spasmodic.

sperma: Gk. = seed or semen, adj.spermatic.

Spermatozoa: = sperm cells. They are the formed male gametes produced by meiosis from cells w/n the walls of seminiferous tubules of the testes. Individual spermatozoa are capable of locomotion due to the presence of a single flagellum.

Spermatic cord (spehr-MAH-tihk kord) a narrow bundle of tissue in the male reproductive system extending from the epididymis to the inguinal canal, consisting of the ductus deferens, cremaster muscle, BVs, lymphatics, nerves, and CT.

sphen- wedge (sven)

sphenoid: adj. Gk. sphen = wedge, and eidos = shape or form; hence the unpaired bone which is wedged into the base of the skull b/n the unpaired frontal and occipital.

sphincter- (sfinkter) tightening associated with a ring of muscle

sphincter: Gk. sphinkter = a tight binder; ie a circular muscle which closes an orifice; adj.- sphincteric.

Spinal cord a long, narrow organ of the CNS that extends through the vertebral canal & connects the PNS with the brain.

Spinal nerve one of 31 pairs of nerves that extend b/n the SC and another part of the body.

spine: Lt. spina = a thorn; a sharp process, or a lay term for the vertebral column; adj.spinous, spinal.

spir- coiled, respiration, breath

sphygm- pressure, pulse

splanchnic: adj. Gk. splanchnon = a viscus or internal organ; hence pertaining to viscera.

Splanchocranium (spl-ANK-noh-KRAY-nee-uhm) that part of the skull containing the facial bones.

Spleen a soft, glandular organ that is part of the lymphatic system & is located in the upper left region of the abdomen behind the stomach.

spleen: Lt. splen = the spleen; hence; adj.- splenic (Lt. - lien).

spongio- description of a skin condition where the keratin layer is thickened and swollen the keratocytes inflated and filled with liquid material due to a defect in Stratum Spingiosum or the prickle layer of the skin

Spongy bone One of2 types of bone tissue, characterized by the presence of spaces filled with red marrow b/n thin bone spicules called trabeculae.

Sputum (SPEW-tum) mucous arising from the lungs - see Phlegm

squama: Lt. = a scale (as of fish or reptile); adj.- squamous.

Squamous (SKWA-muhs) flat, scalelike, square-like.

squamous: adj.Lt. squama = a scale (as of fish or reptile), hence scale-like.

Stage - see grade – measure of the extent of a disease in order to determine management

stapes: Lt. = stirrup; adj.- stapedial, stapedius.

stas- stopped

Static equilibrium the sensation of body position.

steat- fat

stellate: adj. Lt. stella = star.

steno- narrow

stereo- three dimension depth firm solid

stereocilia: Gk. stereos = solid, and cilium = eyelash, hence non-motile microvilli.

sternebra: Gk. sternon = chest or breast, and -bra = from vertebra, the segments of the sternum (these fuse in later life).

sternum: Gk. sternon = chest or breast; adj.- sternal.

Stenosis (STEN-oh-sis) (Gk) narrowing of a duct, BV or other passage.

steth- chest

stoma: Gk. = a mouth.

Stomach (STOH-muhk) a large, hollow organ in the alimentary canal located b/n the oesophagus and small intestine that plays a prominent role in digestion.

stomach: Gk. stomachos = gullet or oesophagus, later applied to the wider part of the digestive tract just below the diaphragm; adj.- gastric.

Stomach mucosa the innermost layer of the stomach wall. It is a mucous membrane that contains numerous gastric glands embedded throughout.

strab- squint

strabismus: Gk. strabismos = squinting; hence, inability to focus both eyes on a given point.

Stratified (STRAH-tif-ide) pertaining to a multiple-layered arrangement of epithelial cells.

stratum: Lt. = a covering sheet, or layer. generally referring to the skin layers.

strepto- twisted

stri- striped, line streak (stry-)

stria: Lt. = furrow, applied to a streak or stripe.

striatum: adj.Lt. striatus = furrowed; hence, corpus striatum, the caudate & lentiform nuclei connected by grey strands which traverse the internal capsule, giving the strands a striated appearance.

Stroma (STROH-mah) supporting bed of cells, CT or matrix upon which or w/n which the structures are placed e.g. the parenchyma.

stroma: Gk. = bed or mattress, the supporting framework of an organ, distinct from its parenchyma.

stroph- twisted

styloid: adj.Gk. stylos = an instrument for writing, and eidos = shape or form; a pencil-like structure.

sub- under, less than partial

subclavian: Lt. sub = under or below, and clavis = a key, hence under the clavicle.

Subcutaneous layer (suhb'-kew-TA-nee-us LA-yehr) the layer of loose CT and adipose tissue deep to the dermis of the skin. (also = hypodermis, and superficial fascia).

subiculum: diminutive of Lt. subix = a support.

sublimis: Lt. = superficial.

Sublingual (suhb-LING-wal) **glands** a pair of salivary glands located in the floor of the mouth deep to the mucous membrane.

Submandibular (sub'-man-DIB-yoo-lah) **glands** a pair of salivary glands located along the inner surface of the jaw in the floor of the mouth. (also = submaxillary glands).

Submucosa (sub'-myoo-KOH-sah) a layer of CT located external to a mucous membrane.

substantia: Lt. = a substance.

Subungal (SUB-ung-gal) under the nail.

succus: Lt. = juice (succus entericus, the secretion of the small intestine).

sud- sweat

Sudoriferous (syoo'-dor-IF-er-us) **gland** an exocrine gland located in the skin that secretes sweat. (also = sweat gland).

sudomotor: Lt. sudor = sweat, and movere = to move, hence

A stimulating the sweat glands.

suf- under

B sulcus: Lt. = a groove.

C **super- over**

D superciliary: adj.Lt. super = above, and cilia = eyelid; hence, pertaining to the eyebrow.

E superficial: adj.Lt. super = above, and facies = surface; hence, nearer the surface.

F **Superficial** (soo'-pehr-FIHSH-ahl) A directional term indicating the location of a part that is toward or nearer to the body surface relative to another ≠ deep.

G H **Superior** (soo-PEER-ee-or) A directional term indicating the location of a part that is nearer to the head region than another. Also called craniad or cephalad.

I J superior: adj.comparative of Lt. superus = above.

supinus- face up

K supination: the act of turning the back of the hand to face posteriorly; verb - supinate ≠ pronate.

L supine: adj.Lt. supinus, recumbent on the back, also, the hand position of the dorsum posteriorly.

M suppuration pus

N **supra- above, over**

O supra: Lt. prefix = superior to.

suprarenal: Lt. supra = above, over, superior to, & ren = the kidney

P sural: adj.Lt. sura = the calf.

Q sustentaculum: Lt. = a support, which sustains; e.g. sustentaculum tali - the ledge on the calcaneus supporting part of the talus.

R S **Suture** (SEW-tjah) the saw-like edge of a cranial bone that serves as a joint b/n bones of the skull; the stitching of 2 opposing edges of tissue.

T suture: Lt. sutura = a seam; the fibrous joints b/n cranial bones.

U **Sweat gland** an exocrine gland located in the skin that secretes sweat. (also = sudoriferous gland).

V **sym- together, union, association**

W sympathetic: Gk. syn = with, and pathos = feeling; hence, the peripheral part of the ANS arising from the thoracolumbar region of the spinal cord and communicates with other nerves.

X **Sympathetic division** (simp'-ah-THEH-tihk dih-VIH-zhuhn) a

Y division of the ANS that functions mainly in stimulating emergency responses (fight or flight).

Z symptom see sign

symphysis: Gk. syn = with, and physis = growth; a joint - bone + **fibrocartilage** + bone generally used for joints in the median plane, often fuse later in life (the symphysis of the mandible is exceptional, the 2 halves fusing before 2 yo).

syn- together, union, association

Synapse (sihn-AHPS) the junction b/n the axon of one neuron & the dendrite or cell body of another neuron.

synapse: Gk. syn = with, and aptein = to join; the zone an impulse passes from one neuron to another.

Synaptic cleft (sihn-AHP-tihk clehft) a part of the synapse that consists of the space b/n neurons or neuron and muscle fibre across which the neurotransmitter must diffuse.

Synaptic end bulb the expanded distal end of a neuron's axon containing numerous synaptic vesicles & mitochondria.

Synaptic terminals the terminal ends of axons where the synapse begins b/n adjacent neurons.

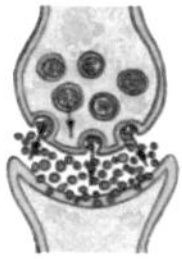

Synaptic vesicles microscopic sacs w/n synaptic end bulbs of axons that store neurotransmitter.

synchondrosis: Gk. syn = with, and chondros = cartilage; a joint - bone + **cartilage** + bone

syncytium: Gk. syn = with, and kytos = cell, a multinucleate mass of protoplasm formed by cells merging as in Giant cells and skeletal muscle cells.

syndesmosis: Gk. syn = with, and desmos = a band; joint - bone + **fibrous tissue** + bone

syndrome: Gk. syn = with, and dromos = running; ie. a group of signs and symptoms, characteristic of a certain pathology.

synergist: Gk. syn = with, and ergon = work; a muscle cooperating with others to produce a certain movement.

synovia: Gk. syn = with, & ovum = egg; the fluid in freely moving joints which resembles egg-white adj. synovial

Synovial fluid the liquid secretion of epithelial cells in the synovial membrane lining a synovial (freely moving) joint, which serves as a lubricant and shock absorber.

Synovial joint (sihn-OH-vee-awl joynt) a type of joint characterized by the presence of a membrane-lined cavity, called the synovial cavity, b/n opposing bones.

systemic (SIS-tem ik) involving the whole body as opposed to local

systole: Gk. = contraction; hence the contraction of cardiac muscle.

A B C D E F G H I J K L M N O P Q R S **T** U V W X Y Z

T

tabe- wasting

tact- touch

taenia: Lt. = a tape or ribbon. AS tenia (TEEN-ih-ah)

tal- ankle

talus: Lt. = ankle-bone; hence, the tortoise-shaped tarsal of the talocrural (ankle) joint.

tars- eyelid , edge of foot

tarsus: Gk. tarsos = a flat surface; the flat part of the foot, later, The bones of the foot behind the metatarsals, adj. tarsal.

Taste buds special sensory organs located primarily on the surface of the tongue & usually embedded within papillae. They contain chemoreceptors, providing the sense of taste or gustation.

taut- same

tect- covering

tectorial: adj.Lt. tectorium = an overlying surface like plaster, a covering or roof.

Tectorial membrane (tehk-TOR-ee-awl MEHM-bran) a thin membrane in the inner ear that projects over the receptor hair cells of the Organ of Corti.

tectum: Lt. = roof; hence the roof of the midbrain.

teg- covering

tegmen: Lt. = covering (c.f. integument = the skin).

tegmentum: Lt. = covering.

tela: Lt. = a web; e.g., a fold of pia mater containing a choroid plexus.

temporal: Lt. tempus = time; the temporal area of the scalp, where grey hair first appears.

Tendon (TEHN-dohn) a band of dense CT that extends from the muscle to attach to a bone.

tendon: Lt. tendo = I stretch out.

tenia: Lt. = a tape or ribbon. AS taenia

tensor: Lt. tensus = stretched; hence a muscle which produces tension.

tentorium: Lt. = tent; tentorium cerebelli.

ter- three

terato- abnormal or monstrous growth

teres: Lt. = rounded, cylindrical.

testicle: Lt. testiculus = the male gonad (see testis).

Testis (TEHS-tihs) one of a pair of male gonads (sex glands) located w/n the scrotum that produces sperm cells & testosterone. pl. - testes.

testis: Lt. testiculus = the male gonad. Lt. testis = a witness. Under Roman law, no man could bear witness (*testify*) unless he possessed both testes. pl. - testes.

Testosterone a steroidal hormone secreted by interstitial cells (cells of Leydig) located w/n the testes. It promotes the development of male secondary sex characteristics & the development of spermatozoa.

terti- third (ter-shi-)

tetralogy: Gk. tetra = four, & logos = discourse, combination of 4 elements e.g. symptoms or defects.

thalamus: Gk. = bedroom - the posterior end of the thalamus is rounded and named pulvinar = cushion.

theca: Gk. theka = a capsule, sheath.

thenar: Gk. = palm of hand; hence, the ball of the thumb.

Thoracic cavity (tho-RAHS-ihk CAHV-ih-tee) the part of the anterior (ventral) body cavity located superior to the diaphragm, which contains the heart, lungs, & mediastinum.

thorax: Gk. = the chest, adj.- thoracic.

Threshold stimulus (THRESH-hold STIH-myoo-luhs) a change in environment.

thrombus: Gk. = a clot.

Thrombocyte (THROHM-bo-sit) the formed elements in blood that play a prominent role in blood clotting. (also = platelets).

Thrombus (THROHM-buhs) a blood clot that has formed in a vein or artery.

thymus: Gk. = sweetbread.

thym- thymus, mind

Thymus (THI-muhs) **gland** a glandular lymphatic organ located superior to the heart that produces T lymphocytes during early childhood, and degenerates by adulthood.

thyroid: Gk. thyreos = shield, & eidos = shape or form; shaped like a shield (shields the glottis).

Thyroid cartilage (THI-royd CAHR-tih-lihj) the largest piece of hyaline cartilage of the larynx. (also = the Adam's apple).

Thyroid gland (THI-royd) an endocrine gland located on the anterior side of the neck that secretes hormones involved in growth, metabolism, and maintaining calcium levels in the blood.

tibia: Lt. = the shin-bone, adj.- tibial.

Tissue (TIH-shoo) a group of similar cells that combine to form a common function.

A B C D E F G H I J K L M N O P Q R S **T** U V W X Y Z

Tongue (tuhng) the muscular organ of the digestive system that is anchored to the floor of the mouth and wall of the pharynx. It plays major roles in swallowing and speech formation.

Tonsil (TOHN-sihl) a small organ of the lymphatic system that consists of an aggregation of fixed lymphocytes & CT embedded in a mucous membrane. There are 3 pairs (pharyngeal, palatine & lingual), all of which play a role in the immune response.

tonsil: Lt. tonsilla = tonsil (e.g., palt.e tonsil).

Tooth a bony structure projecting from the maxilla or mandible that provides for the grinding, or mechanical digestion, of food particles.

top- on the surface, to place

Tophus (TOE-fus) collection of urate crystals in gout

tors- twisted bulge

torus: Lt. = a bulge.

Trabecula (traw-BEHK-yoo-lar) a thin plate of bone within spongy bone tissue. (also = a band of supportive CT extending to the interior of an organ from its outer wall as in the spleen or the breast).

trabecula: diminutive of Lt. trabs = a beam; hence the supporting fibres of a structure.

Trachea (TRA-kee-aw) an organ of the respiratory system consisting of a long tube supported by semi-rings of cartilage extending from the pharynx to the bronchi.

trachea: Gk. tracheia = rough, referring to its corrugations.

tract: Lt. tractus = an elongated strand of wool or dough; hence a pathway for nerve fibres.

tragus: Lt. = goat, because of the beard-like tuft of hair on its internal aspect.

trans- across

Transitional epithelium a type of epithelial tissue characterized by its ability to expand in size and recoil, giving the organs it lines a feature of elasticity. Transitional epithelium forms the inner lining of the urinary bladder and ureters

transverse: perpendicular to the long axis = horizontal.

Transverse colon the segment of the colon that extends across the body from its union with the ascending colon (Left) to its union with the descending colon (Left).

trapezium: Gk. trapezion = a trapezium - a quadrilateral with 2 sides parallel.

trapezius: Gk. trapezion = a trapezium - a quadrilateral with 2 sides parallel; hence, trapezius muscle, the diamond-shape of both trapezii muscles together.

trapezoid: Gk. trapezion = a trapezium - a quadrilateral with 2 parallel sides, resembling a trapezium.

Trauma (TRAW-mah) Gk. injury, wound physical or psychological.

tri- three (try)

Triad when pertaining to the liver, a triad is a combination of 3 structures that can be observed in a cross-sectional microscopic view. They include branches of the hepatic portal vein, hepatic artery, and bile duct. When pertaining to skeletal muscle, a triad refers to a T tubule and two cisternae of the sarcoplasmic reticulum.

triad: from Lt. tres = 3.

triceps: Lt. tres = 3, & caput = head; hence a 3-headed muscle.

tricho (TRIK-oh) hair

trigeminal: Lt. trigeminus = triplets; hence, cranial nerve V, with 3 large divisions.

trigone: Lt. trigonum = a triangle.

triquetral: Lt. triquetrus = 3-cornered.

triticea: Lt. triticum = a grain of wheat; hence, the tiny cartilage in the lateral thyrohyoid ligament.

trocho- round

trochanter: Gk. = a runner; the bony landmark, the greater trochanter, moves obviously in running.

trochlea: Gk. trochilia = a pulley.

trop- turn, change

troph- nutrition

truncus: Lt. = trunk (of a tree).

tube: origin unknown

tubule: little tube

tuber: Lt. tuber = a swelling or lump. (see protuberance)

Tubercle (TEW-ber-cl) a small process or bump generally on a bone.

tubercle: Lt. diminutive of tuber, a small prominence, usually bony. (smaller than a tuberosity).

tuberculum: Lt. diminutive of tuber, a small prominence, usually bony

tuberosity: Lt. tuber = a swelling or lump, usually large & rough (larger than a tubercle).

tunica: Lt. = shirt; hence a covering.

Tunica externa (TEW-nih-kah eks-TEHRN-ah) the outermost layer of a tubular BV wall. (also = the tunica adventitia and the serosa, it is composed of CT and in larger vessels smaller BVs the vasa vasorium).

Tunica intima (TEW-nih-kah IHN-tih-mah) the innermost, or deepest, layer of a tubular BV. (also = the tunica interna, it is composed of a layer of simple squamous epithelium (endothelium) and a BM of CT.

Tunica media (TEW-nih-kah ME-de-ah) the middle layer forming the wall of a tubular BV. The tunica media is composed of smooth muscle tissue, and may contain elastic fibres.

turbinate: Lt. turbo = a child's (spinning) top; hence shaped like a top. An old term for the nasal conchi.

Tympanic membrane (tihm-PAHN-ihk MEHM-bran) a thin membrane b/n the external auditory canal & the tympanic cavity, separating the external ear from the middle ear. (also = the eardrum).

tympanum: Lt. = a drum.

U

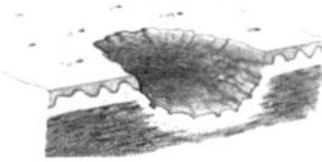

Ulcer (UL-ser) Lt ulcus = wound, sore, hence lack of continuity on a surface must penetrate al the layers of the skin.

ulna: Lt. = elbow or arm; hence, the medial bone of the forearm.

ultra- beyond, in excess

umbilicus: Lt. = the navel.

umbo: Lt. = the boss on the centre of a shield, umbo of tympanic membrane.

uncinate: Lt. uncinatus = hooked.

uncus: Lt. = hook; adj.- uncinate.

ungu- nails (UNG-gu)

ungual: pertaining to Lt. unguis = finger-nail.

uni- first one

urachus: Gk. ouron = urine, and echein = to hold, the canal connecting the foetal bladder and umbilicus.

Ureter (YEW-reh-tehr) a long, narrow muscular tube extending from the kidney to the urinary bladder & transports urine using gravity and peristalsis.

ureter: Gk. oureter = passage from kidney to bladder.

Urethra (yew-REE-thrah) a tube extending from the urinary bladder to the exterior that carries urine in females and urine and semen in males.

urethra: Gk. ourethra = passage from bladder to exterior.

uterus: Lt. = womb.

Urtica = hive - local swelling on the skin.

utricle: diminutive of Lt. uterus = womb.

Urinary bladder (yew'-rih-NAR-ee BLAH-dehr) a hollow muscular organ located at the floor of the pelvic cavity that temporarily stores urine.

Uterine tube (YEW-tehr-ihn toob) One of 2 tubes that transport ova from the ovaries to the uterus in the female reproductive system. (also = the fallopian tubes or oviducts).

Uterus (YEW-tehr-uhs) a hollow muscular organ in the female reproductive system that serves as a site of embryo implantation, development and menstruation.

uvea: Lt. uva = grape. The pigmented vascular layer of the eyeball (iris, ciliary body and choroid).

uvula: diminutive of Lt. uva = grape.

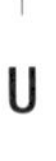

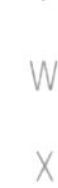

V

Vagina (vaj-EYE-nah) a tubular, muscular organ of the female reproductive system extending b/n the vulva & the uterus.

vagina: Lt. = sheath; hence, invagination is the acquisition of a sheath by pushing inwards into a membrane, and evagination is similar but produced by pushing outwards.

vagus: Lt. = wandering; hence, cranial nerve X, which leaves the head and neck to traverse the thorax & upper part of the abdomen

valgus: Lt. = bow-legged.

vallate: Lt. vallatus = walled; hence, the large papillae on the tongue which are depressed below the surface & surrounded by a groove which is itself bounded by a wall.

vallecula: diminutive of Lt. vallis = a fossa.

Valve a membranous flap composed of CT and usually lined by a layer of epithelium which directs the flow of fluid in one direction.

valve: Lt. valva = the segment of a folding-door.

valvula: diminutive of Lt. valva.

varicocoele: Lt. varix = vein and Gk. kele = tumor, hernia, a varicose condition of the veins of the pampiniform plexus.

Varix (VAR-ix) : Lt. dilated vein.

varus: Lt. = knock-kneed.

vas: Lt. = vessel (plural = vasa).

Vas deferens also = the ductus deferens. It is a tube extending between the epididymis and the urethra in the male that conveys spermatozoa during ejaculation.

Vascular (VAHS-kyoo-lawr) Pertaining to or containing BVs.

vascular: Lt. vasculum, diminutive of vas; hence, pertaining to BVs.

Vein (vayn) a BV that transports blood from body tissues to the heart.

vein: Lt. vena; adj.- venous. (veen-us)

velum: Lt. = curtain; veli = of a curtain.

ven- vein

Venipuncture (VEEN-EE–punc-tewr) puncturing of a vein – (in order to take a blood sample)

venter: Lt. = belly; hence, ventral, pertaining to the belly side.

Ventral (VEN-tral) a directional term describing the location of a part nearer to the anterior or front side of the body relative to another. (also = anterior).

Ventral root the motor branch of a spinal nerve that connects with the SC.

Ventricle (VEN-trih-kuhl) one of the 2 inferior, highly muscular chambers of the heart that push blood into major arteries during their contraction.

ventricle: diminutive of Lt. venter = a small belly.

Venule (VEN-yewl) a small vein that collects deoxygenated blood from a capillary network and conveys it to a larger vein.

vermiform: Lt. vermis = a worm, and forma = shape; hence, worm-shaped.

Vermiform appendix (VEHR-mih-form aw-PEHN-dihks) a small, closed-end tube extending from the caecum of the large intestine.

Vermis (VEHR-mihs) the central constricted part of the cerebellum that separates the 2 cerebellar hemispheres.

vermis: Lt. = worm; hence, the segmented median part of the cerebellum.

verruca: wart

vertebra: Lt. verto = I turn; one of the movable bones of the VC.

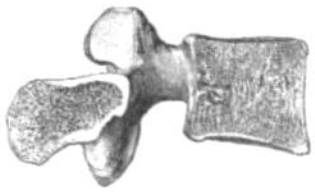

Vertebral canal (VEHR-teh-brahl kah-NAHL) a cavity extending through the vertebral column that is formed by the vertebral foramina of each vertebra, through which extends the SC.

Vertebral column The skeleton of the back that is composed of 26 vertebrae and associated tissues. (also = the backbone, spine, or spinal column).

vertex: Lt. = summit; hence the highest point on the skull.

vertical: perpendicular (at a right angle) to the horizontal.

vesic- to do with the baldder

vesica: Lt. = bladder, adj.- vesical.

Vesicle (VEHS-ih-kuhl) a small sac containing a fluid. In the cell, it is a membranous sac w/n the cytoplasm which contains cellular products or waste materials.

vesicle: diminutive of Lt. vesica = bladder, hence a little bladder

vesicula: diminutive of Lt. vesica = bladder; seminal vesicle.

Vestibular membrane (vehs-TIHB-yew-lahr MEHM-brayn) a thin membrane inside the membranous labyrinth of the inner ear.

Vestibule (VEHS-tih-byewl) a small space that opens into a larger cavity or canal. A vestibule is found in the inner ear, mouth, nose, and vagina.

vestibule: Lt. vestibulum = entrance hall.

vibrissa: Lt. vibrare = to vibrate; hence, the hairs in the nasal vestibule which vibrate in the air.

Villus (VIHL-luhs) a small, fingerlike projection of the small intestinal wall containing CT, BVs, and a lymphatic vessel, and which functions in the absorption of nutrients. pl. - villi.

villus: Lt. a hair; hence, a vascular, hair-like process, usually projecting from a mucous surface.

vincula: Lt. = fetters (sing. - vinculum); delicate vascular synovial bands passing to the digital tendons.

Visceral (VIHS-er-ahl) pertaining to the internal components (mainly the organs) of a body cavity; pertaining to the outer surface of an internal organ ≠ parietal.

visceral: adj.Lt. viscus = an internal organ.

Visceral peritoneum (VIHS-er-ahl per'-ih-toh-NEE-uhm) a serous membrane covering the surfaces of abdominal organs.

Visceral pleura (VIHS-er-ahl PLEW-rah) a serous membrane covering the outer surface of each lung.

viscus: Lt. = an internal organ, plural - viscera, adj.- visceral.

vital: Lt. vita = life.

vitelline: Lt. vitellus = yolk.

vitreous: Lt. vitreus = glassy.

Vitreous humor (VIH-tree-uhs HYEW-mahr) a mass of gelatinous material located w/n the eyeball in the posterior cavity located b/n the lens and the retina. (also = vitreous body).

vivi- alive

vocal: adj. Lt. vox = voice.

volar: pertaining to the palm or the sole of the foot

volv- turn

vomer: Lt. = plough-share; hence, the bone of the nasal septum which is split in two at its upper edge.

vulgar: Lt vulgaris = usual; common, plentiful.

vulva: Lt. = the external female genitalia.

W

White matter a type of NT composed mainly of the myelinated axons of neurons.
White pulp one of the 2 interior areas of the spleen (see red pulp). White pulp is composed of lymphocytes, monocytes and macrophages suspended on a stroma of reticular fibres. It provides immunological and phagocytic functions in the spleen.

X

xanth- yellow
xen- different
xero- dry

xiphoid: Gk. xiphos = a sword, and eidos = shape or form; hence, sword-shaped.

Y

Yellow marrow a collection of fat storage (adipose) & other tissues found w/n the medullary cavities of bones.

Z

Zona (ZOH-nah) an area smaller than a region in an organ as in the adrenal gland.

zona: Lt. = a belt; hence, a circular band.
zonule: diminutive of zona.
zoster: Lt girdle.

zyg- yoke (z-eye-g)

zygoma: Gk. zygon = yoke; hence, the bone joining the maxillary, frontal, temporal & sphenoid bones.

zygomatic: adj.Gk. zygon = yoke; the bone joining the maxillary.

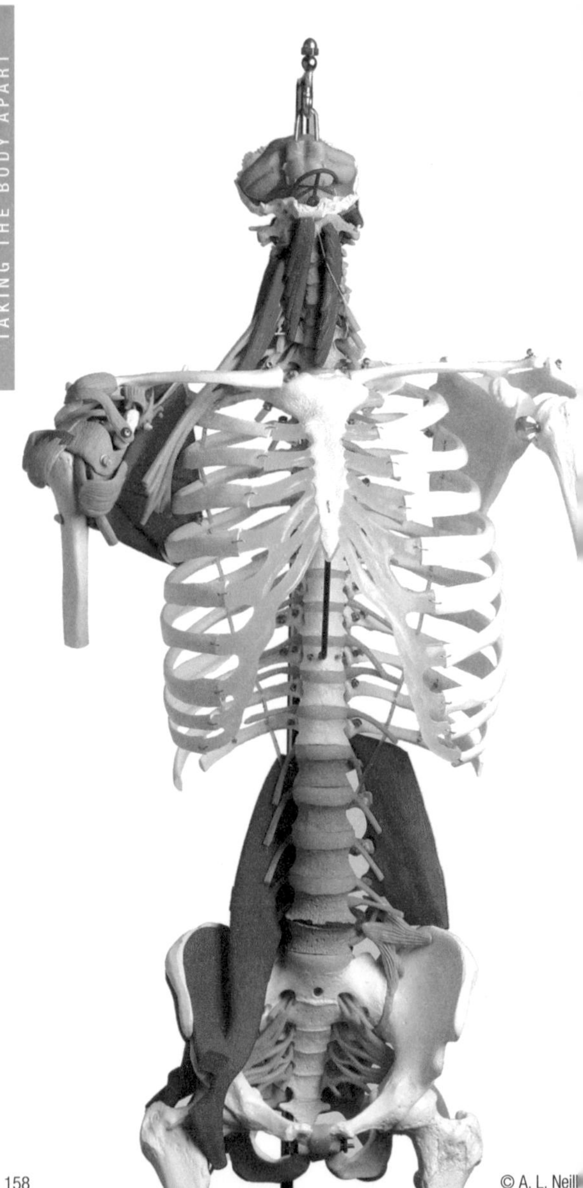

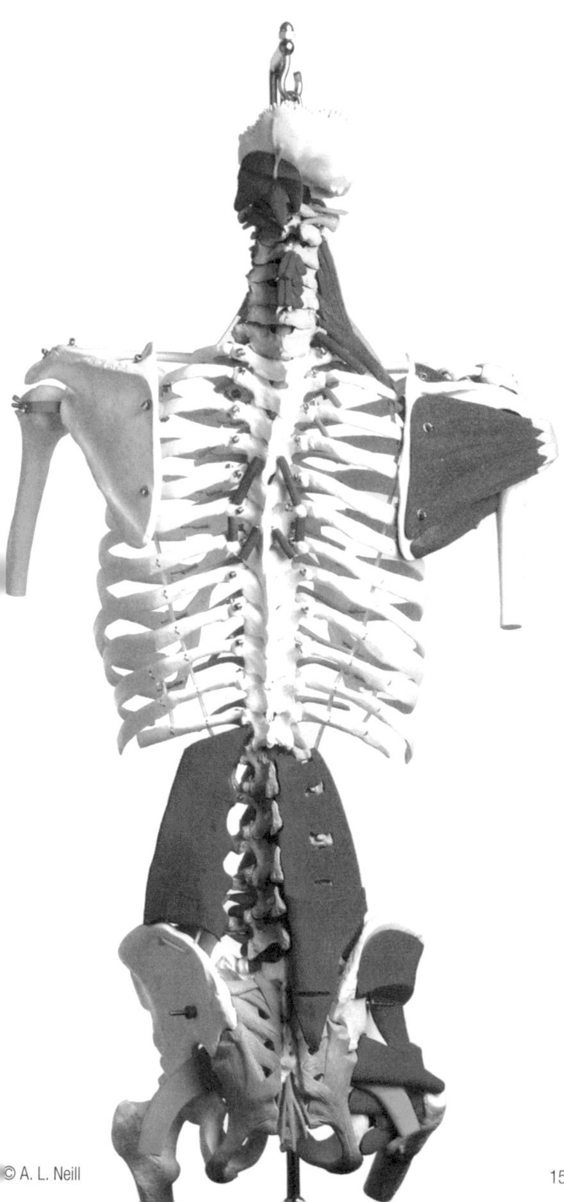

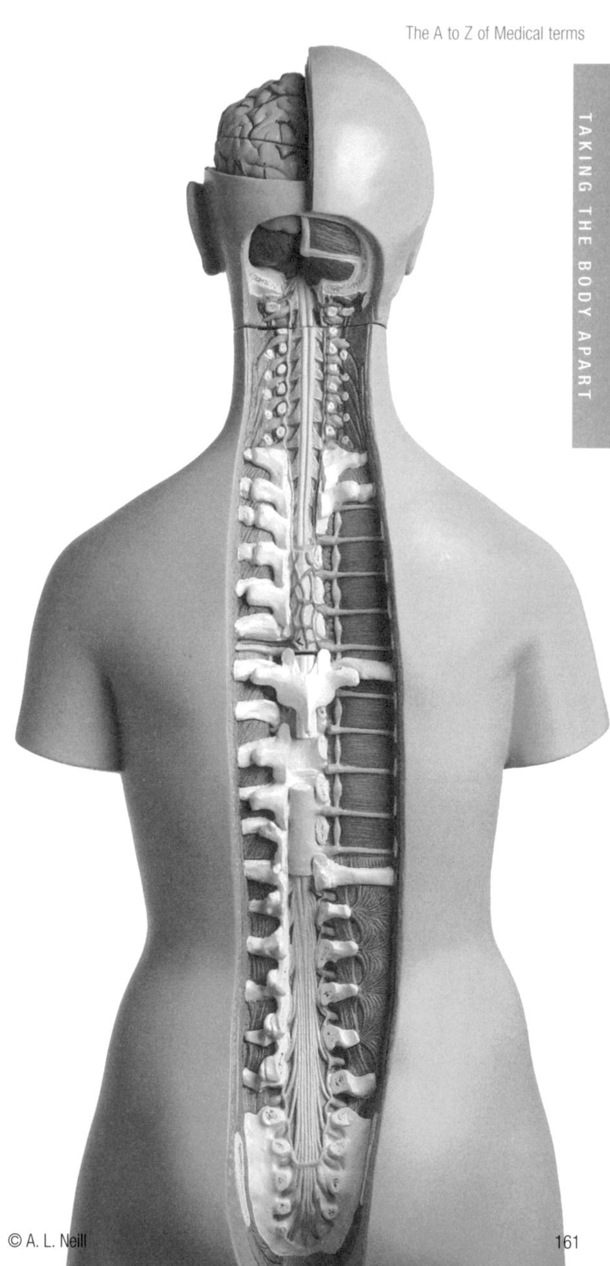

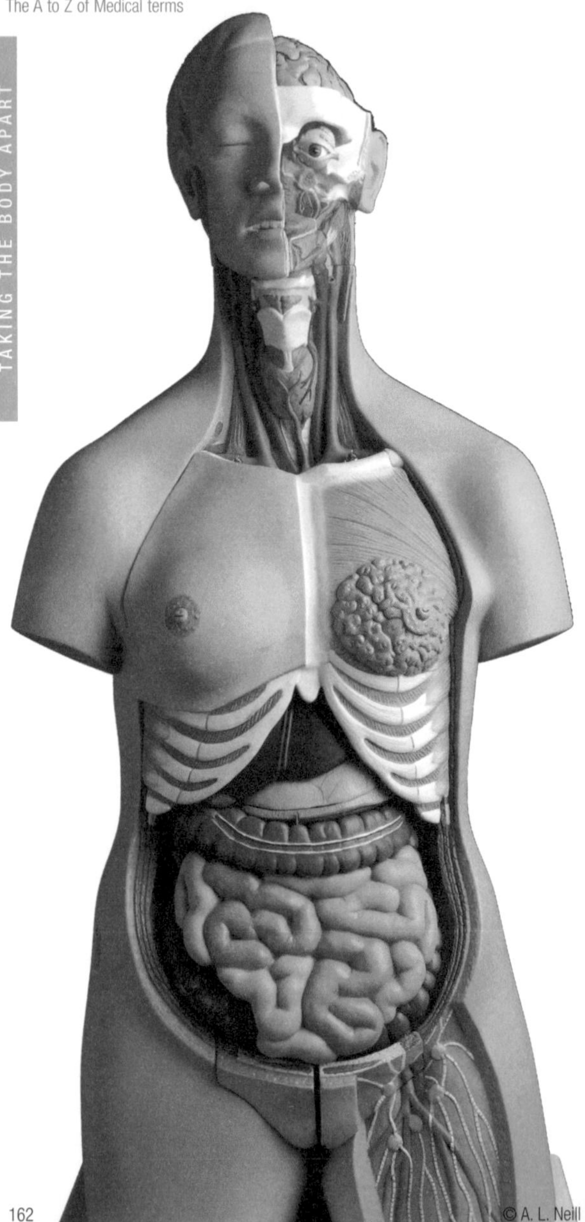

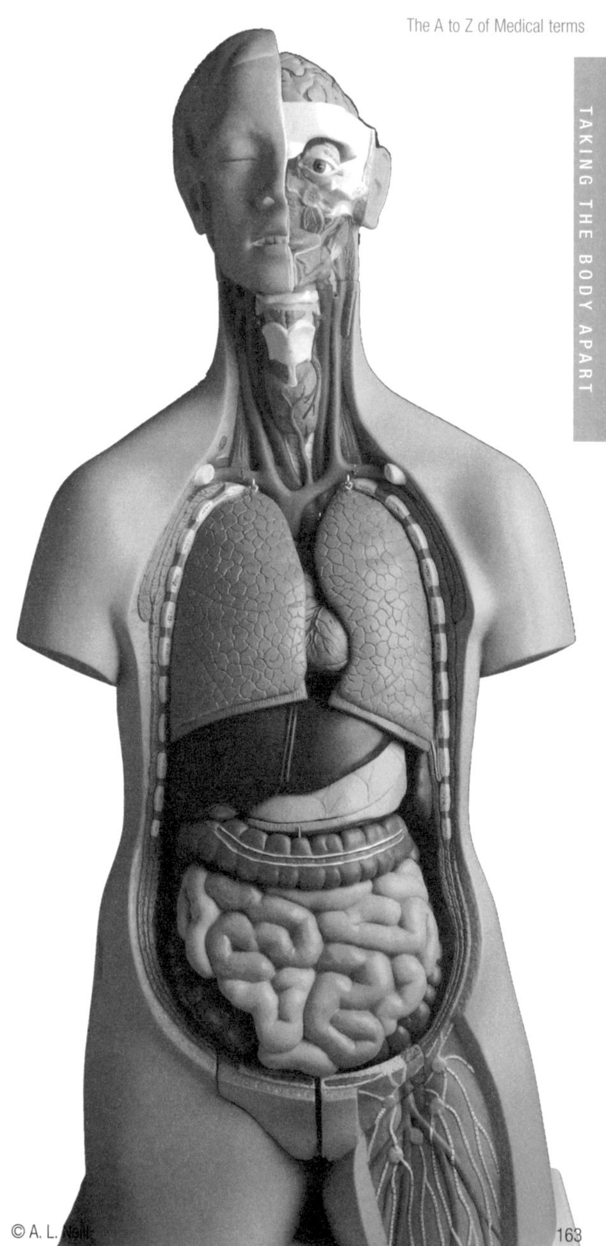

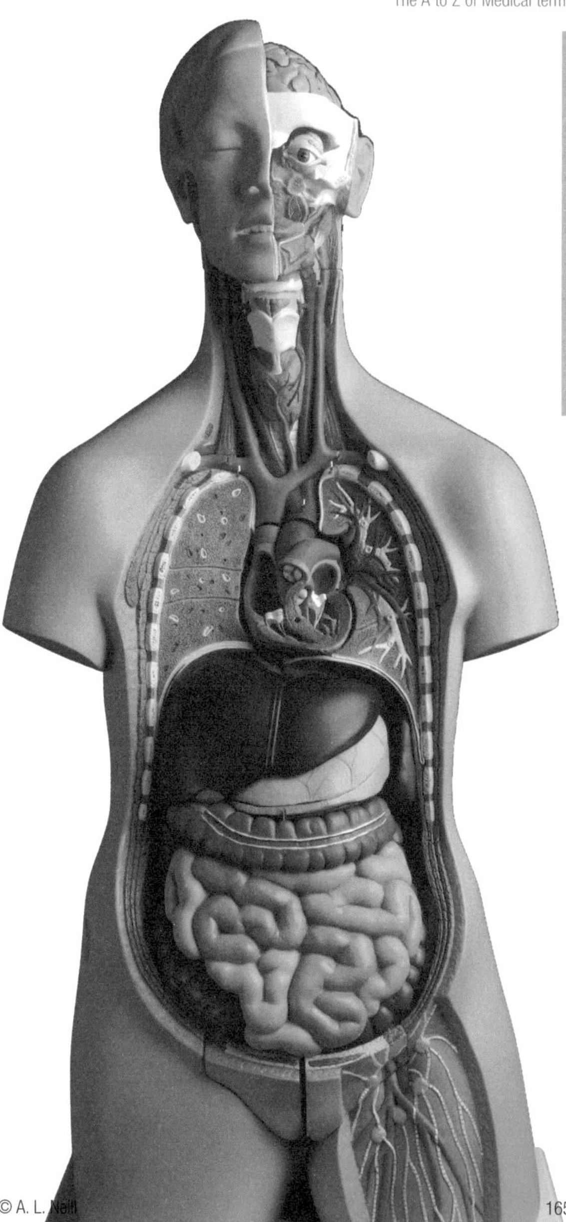

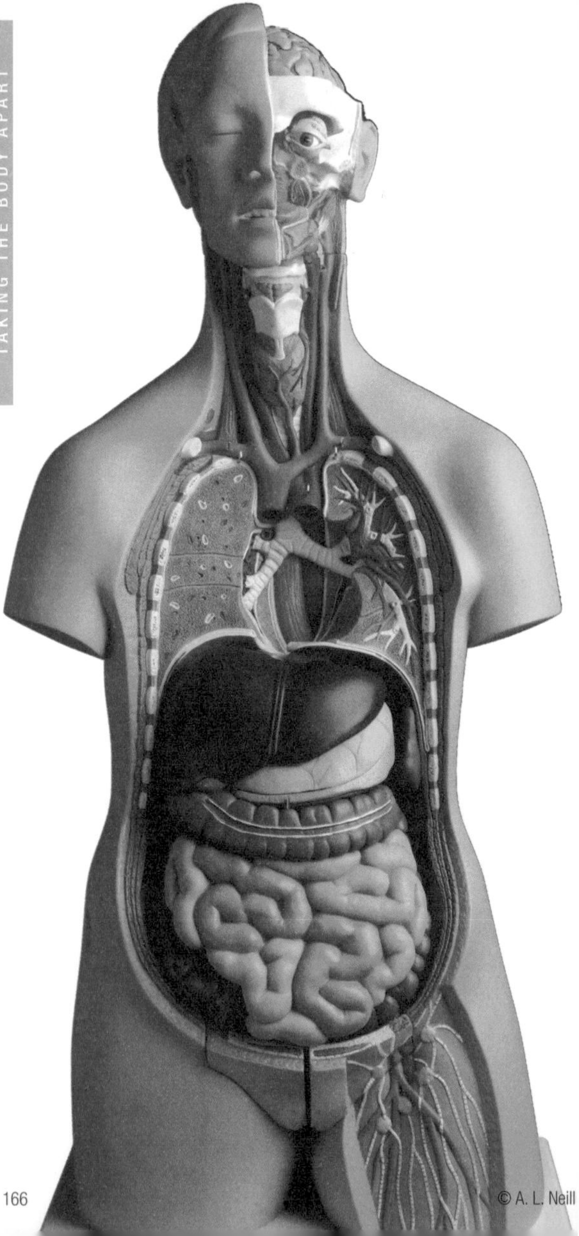

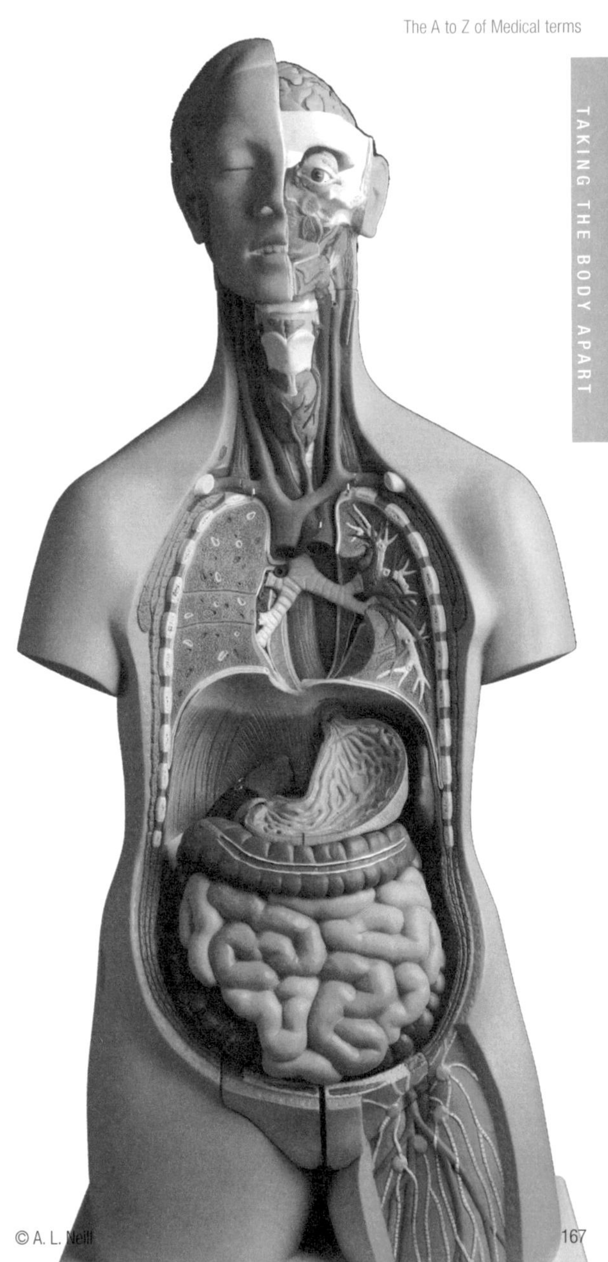

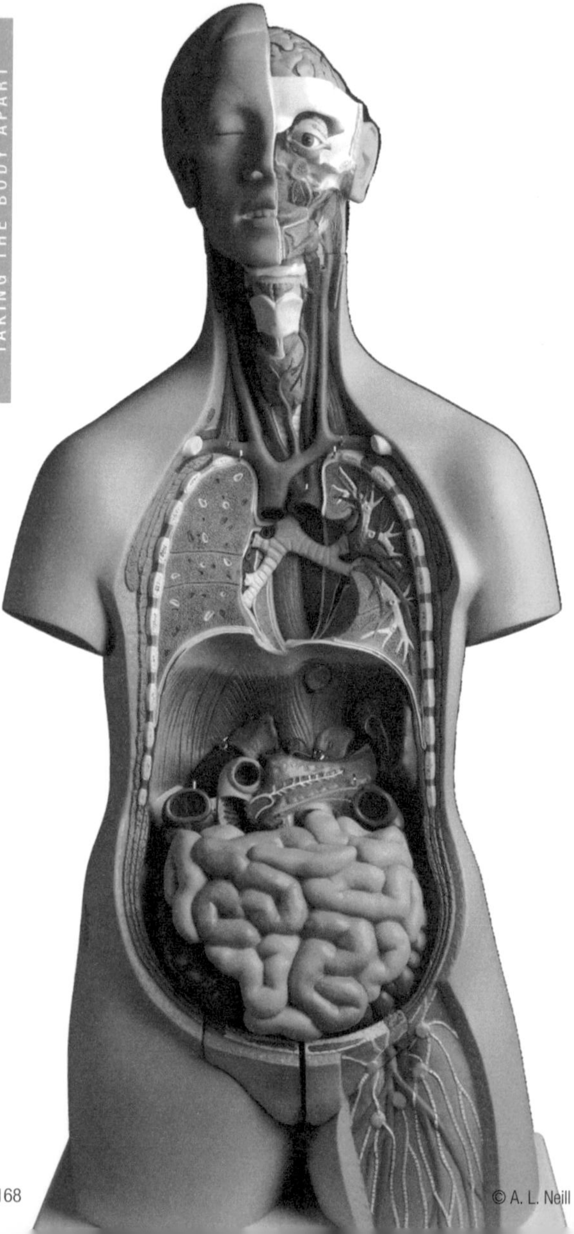

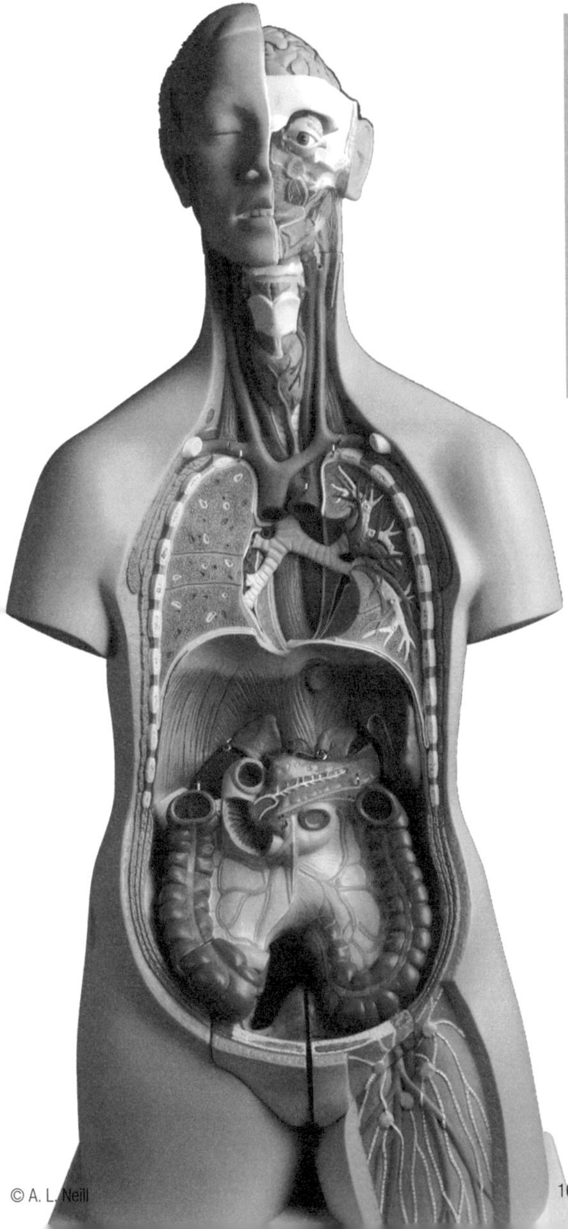

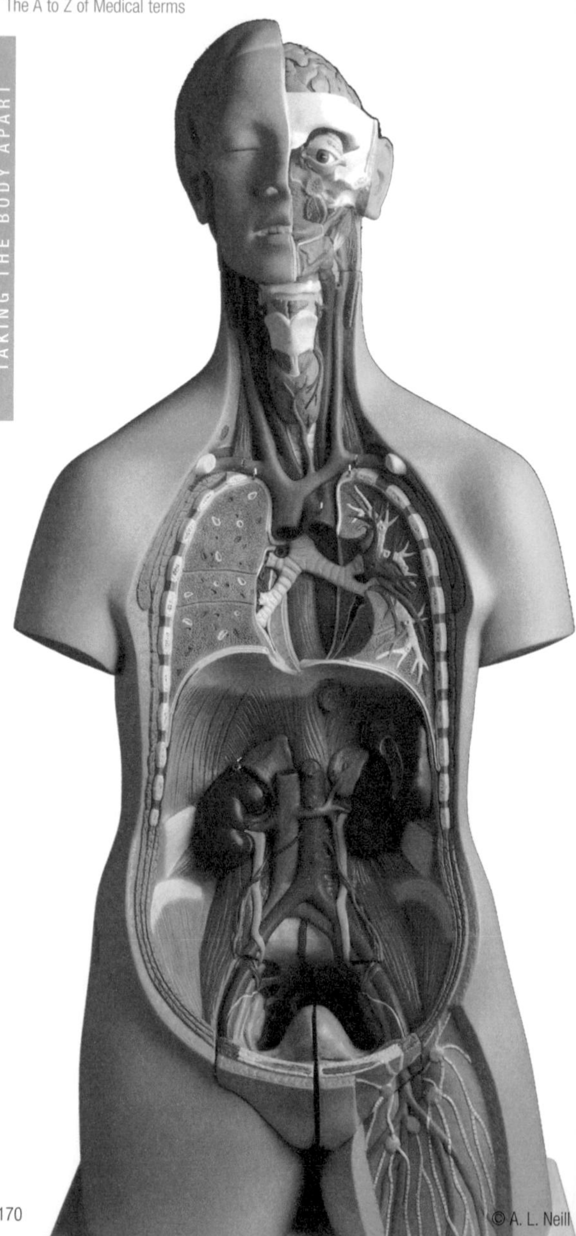

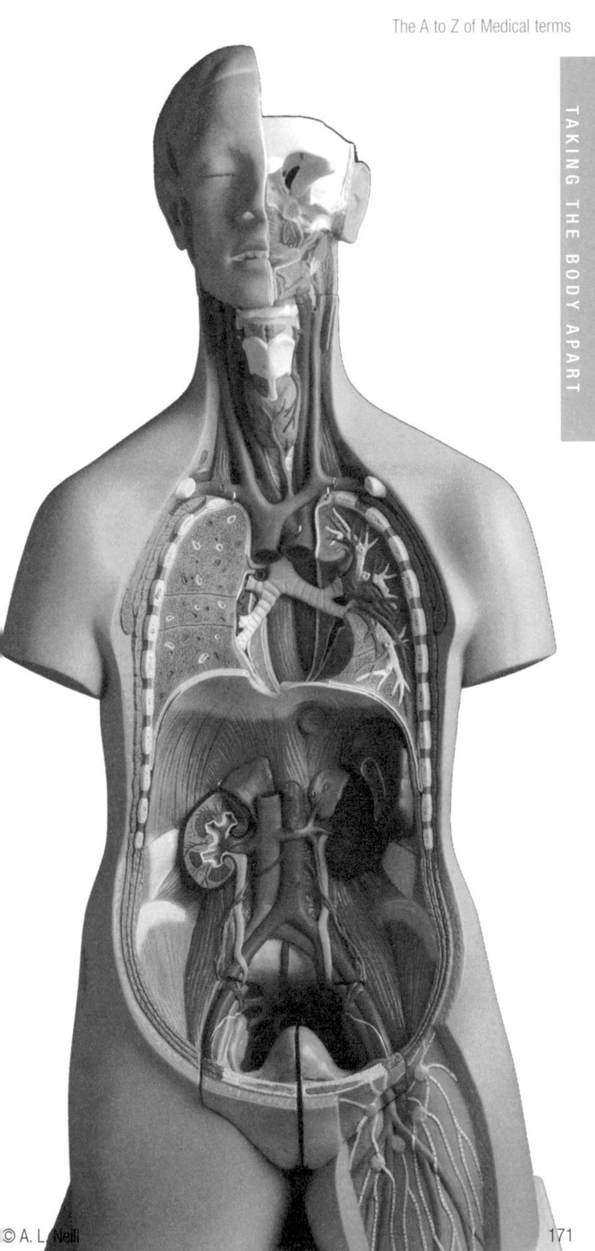

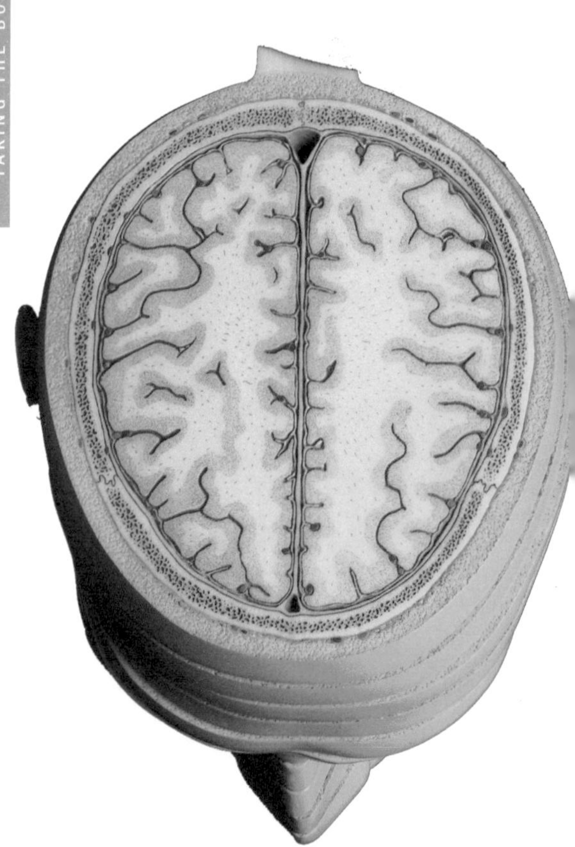

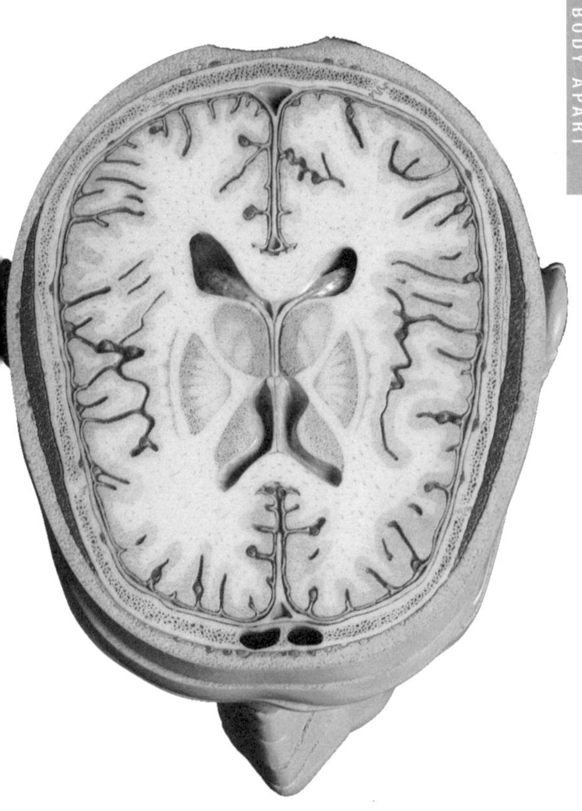

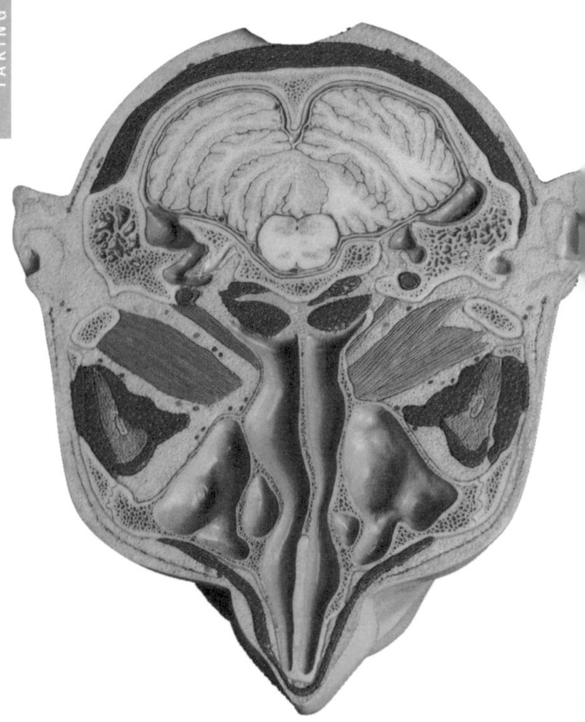

Surface Anatomy and Surface Markers

HORIZONTAL

- C1= the Hard palate
- C2 = free margin of the upper teeth
- C2/3 = Hyoid bone
- C4 = upper level of the Thyroid cartilage
- C6 = Cricoid cartilage
- T1 = vertebra prominens
- T7 = Thoracic plane
- T9/10 = Sterno-Xiphoid plane
- L1 = Transpyloric plane
- L3 = Subcostal plane
- L3/4 = Umbilical plane
- L5 = intertubercular plane

VERTICAL

- Lateral vertical line = through the lateral extremity of the 9th costal cartilage.
- Median vertical plane / Sagittal plane = through the centre of the body and vertebral column
- Midclavicular line = through the middle of the clavicle

INTERSECTION POINTS

- Lateral vertical lines + Transpyloric plane = Lateral central points
- Median line + L1 = central point

9 ABDOMINAL REGIONS - intersection of the lateral vertical planes and the transpyloric and the intertubercular planes

Right Hypochondriac	Epigastric	Left Hypochondriac
Right Lumbar	Umbilical	Left Lumbar
Right Iliac	Hypogastric	Left Iliac

***For more details see** The A to Z of Surface Anatomy.*

Anatomical Planes and Relations

This is the anatomical position.

A= Anterior Aspect from the front Posterior Aspect from the back used interchangeably with ventral and dorsal respectively
B= Lateral Aspect from either side
C= Transverse / Horizontal plane
D= Midsagittal plane = Median plane; trunk moving away from this plane = lateral flexion or lateral movement moving into this plane medial movement; limbs moving away from this direction = abduction; limbs moving closer to this plane = adduction
E= Coronal plane
F= Median

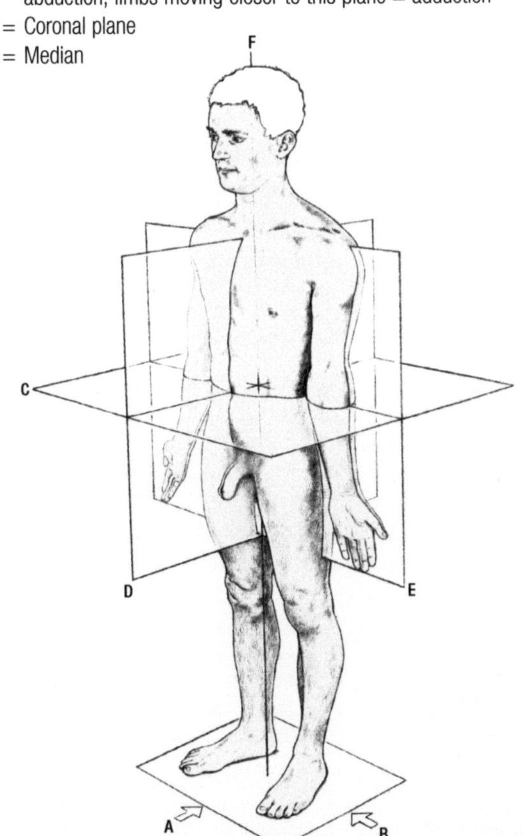

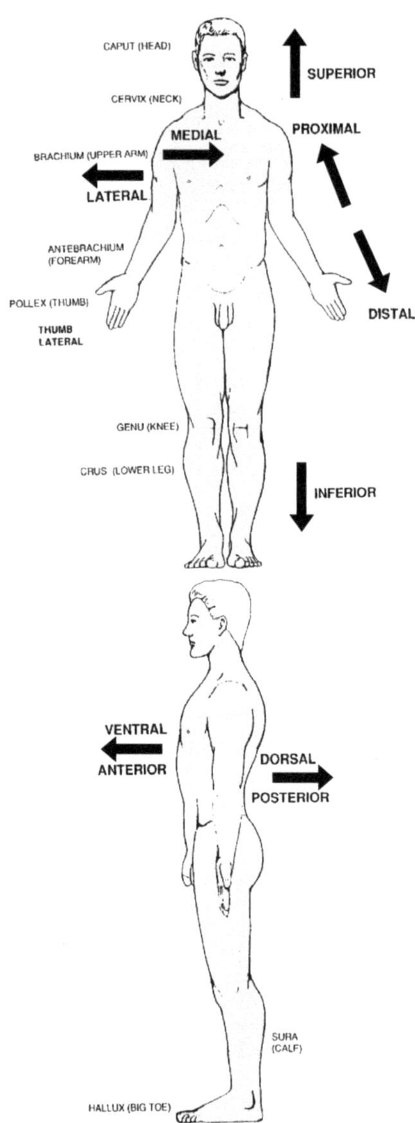
CAPUT (HEAD)
SUPERIOR
CERVIX (NECK)
MEDIAL
PROXIMAL
BRACHIUM (UPPER ARM)
LATERAL
ANTEBRACHIUM
(FOREARM)
POLLEX (THUMB)
THUMB
LATERAL
DISTAL
GENU (KNEE)
CRUS (LOWER LEG)
INFERIOR
VENTRAL
ANTERIOR
DORSAL
POSTERIOR
SURA
(CALF)
HALLUX (BIG TOE)

Anatomical Movements - Back

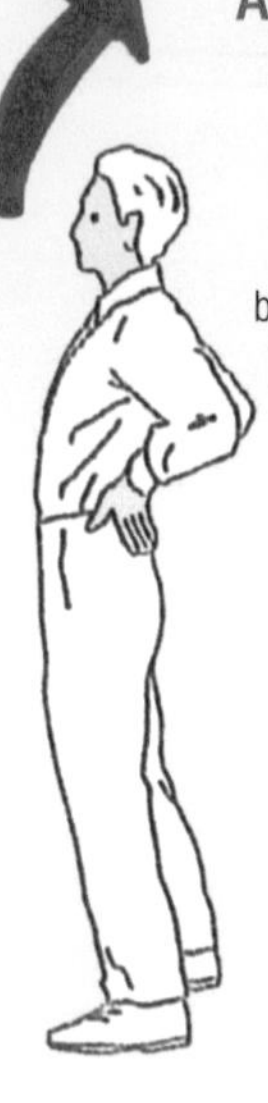

back extension / hyperextension
note the back muscles are
contracting

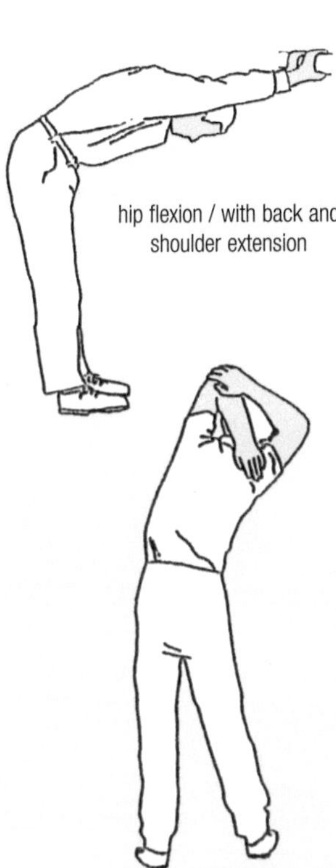

hip flexion / with back and
shoulder extension

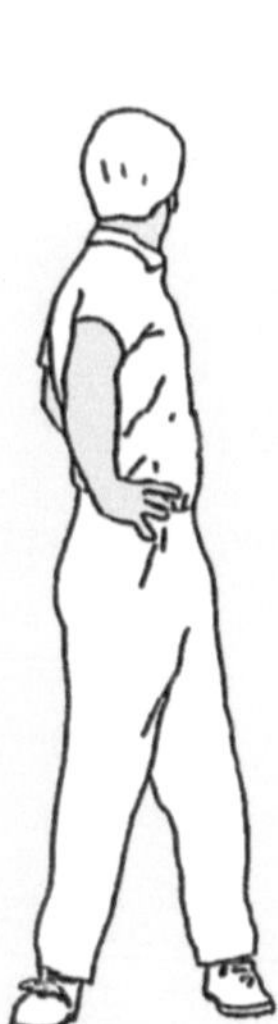

back rotation

back lateral flexion shoulder
extension and elbow flexion

Anatomical Movements - Foot & hand

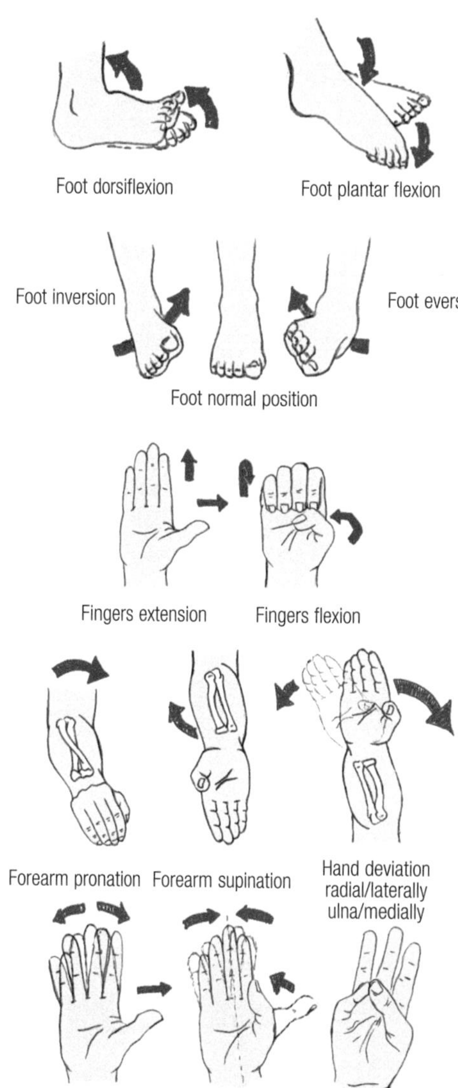

Foot Movements

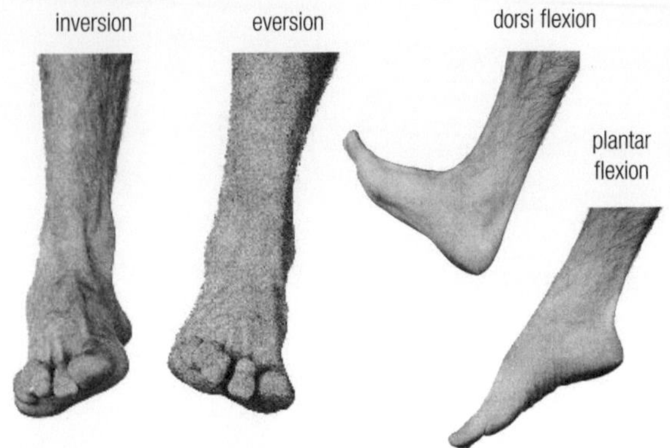

Hand Movements & Grips

The hand & wrist may be involved in a huge range of different grips & fine specialized movements calling upon a combination of muscles to allow for the precision of the actions.

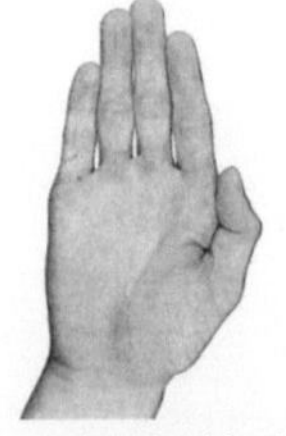

Finger thumb adduction
Dorsal Interossei

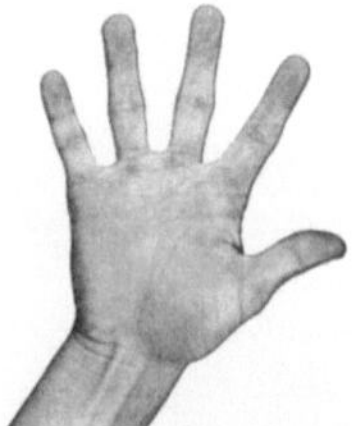

Finger thumb abduction
Palmar Interossei

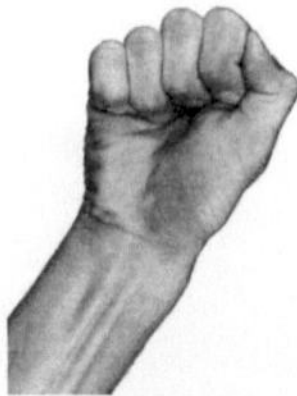

Finger thumb flexion
FDP, FPL

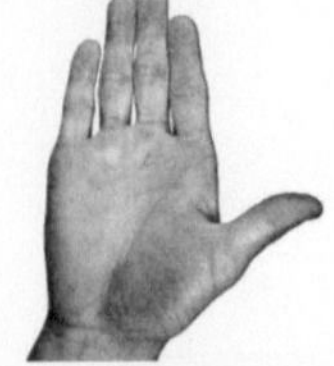

Finger thumb extension ant. dorso-lat *(anat snuff box) ED, EP*

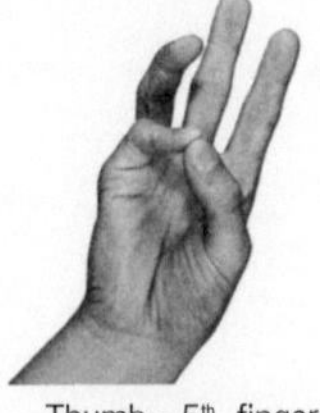

Thumb - 5th finger opposition *TE, HE, OP*

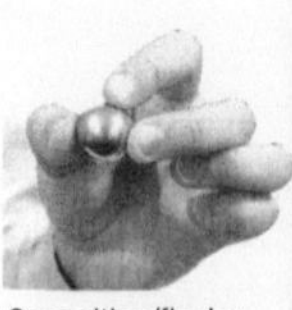

Opposition/flexion
Carpal curve for precision grip

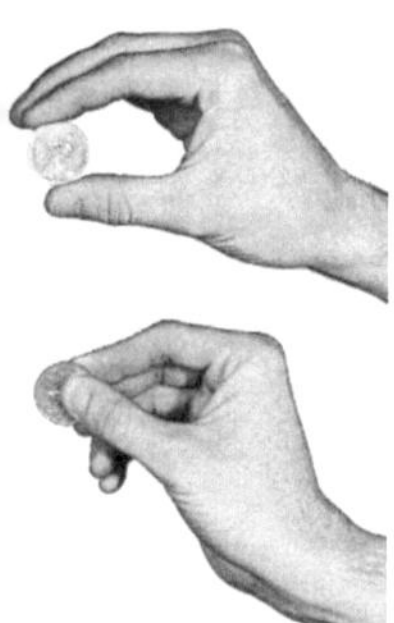

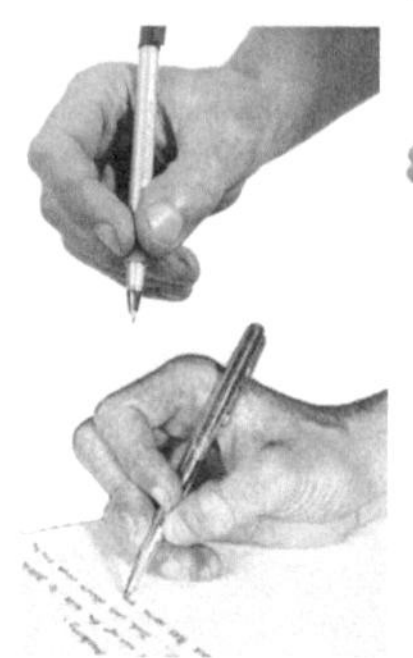

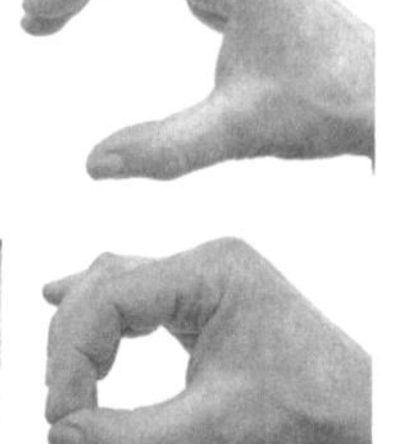

Thumb index – precision grip *TE, HE, OP*

Thumb fingers - ± intrinsic hand muscles writing grip - precision *interossei*

Open grip, Pinch lat.

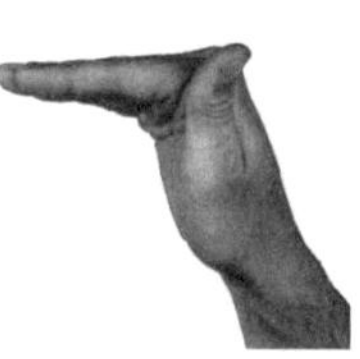

Finger extension - hand flexion *Lumbricles*

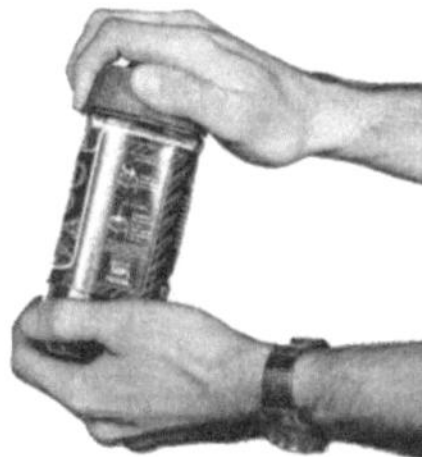

Hands coordinate in 2 handed procedures – unscrewing

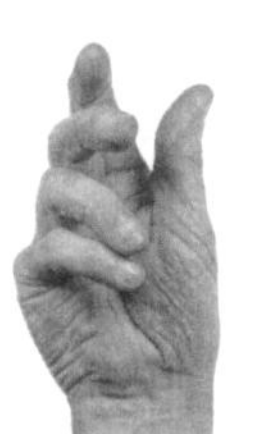

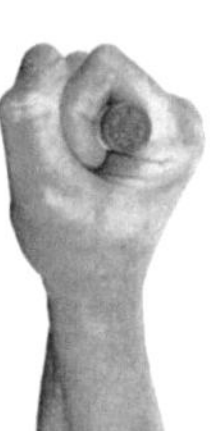

Power grips making use of friction - finger tips, PB HE+ TE for additional grip also boney curves - carpal curve shape of the phalanges

Practical holds demonstrating power grip variations

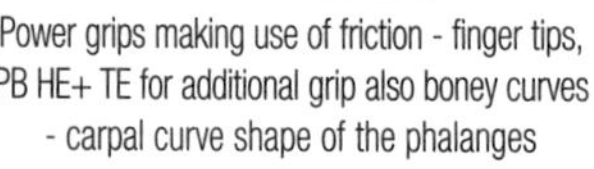

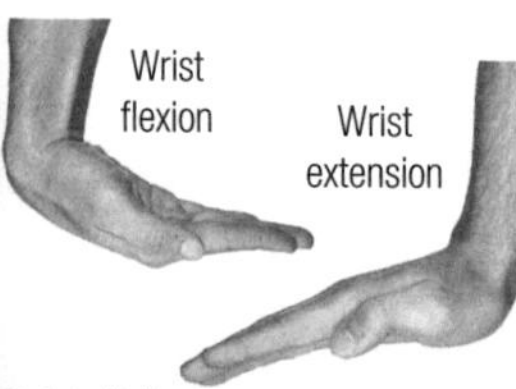

Wrist flexion

Wrist extension

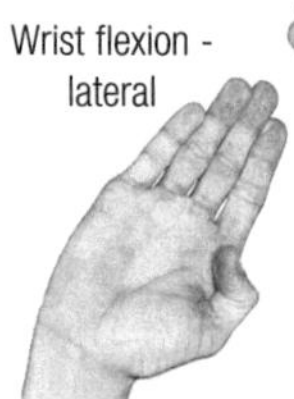

Wrist flexion - lateral

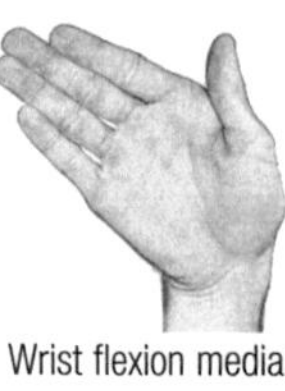

Wrist flexion medial

Anatomical Movements - Head & Neck

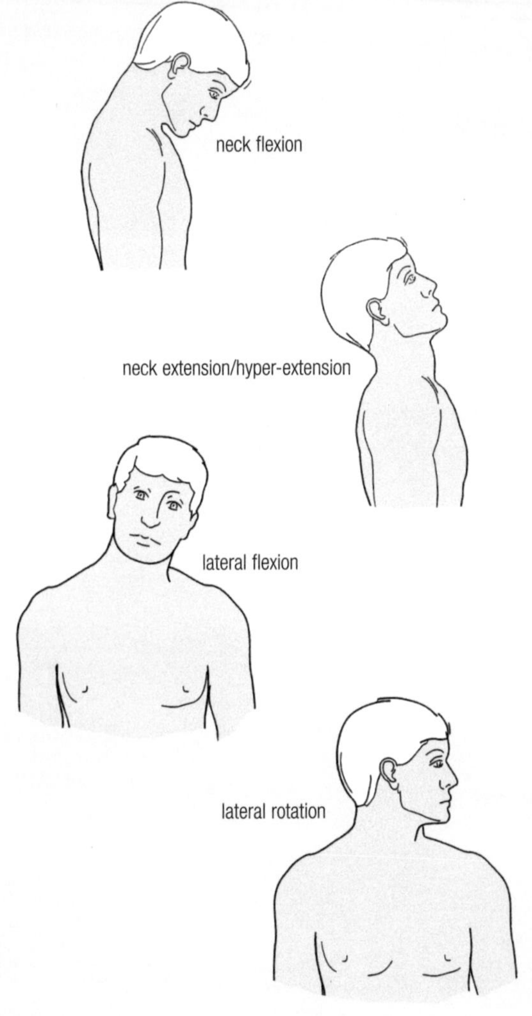

note: extension of the neck is in the normal anatomical position

Anatomical Movements - Lower limb & Hip

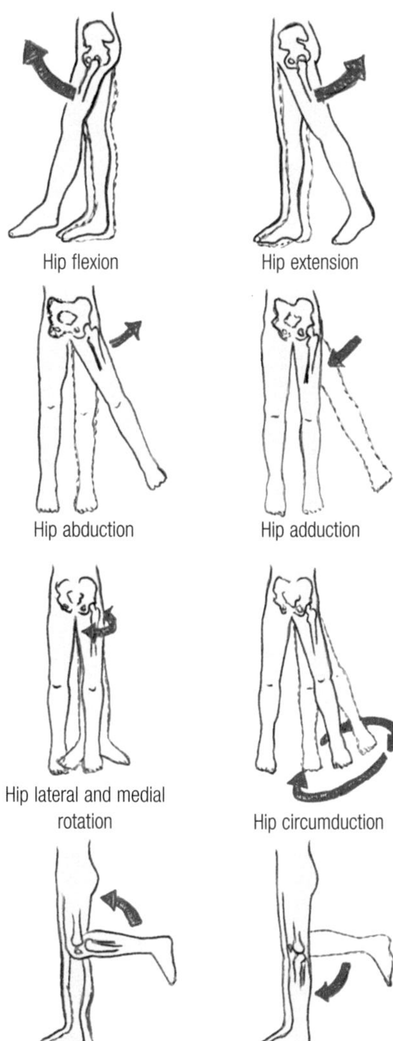

Hip flexion

Hip extension

Hip abduction

Hip adduction

Hip lateral and medial rotation

Hip circumduction

Knee flexion

Knee extension

Anatomical Movements - Upper limb & shoulder

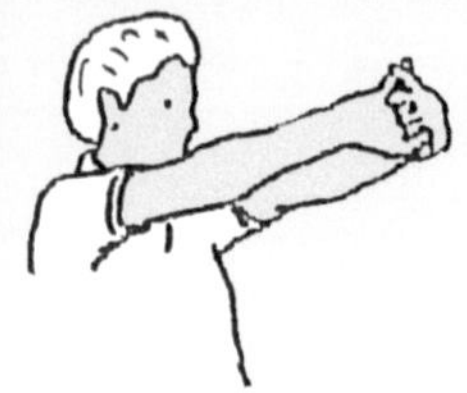

arm extension in sagittal plane / shoulder movement

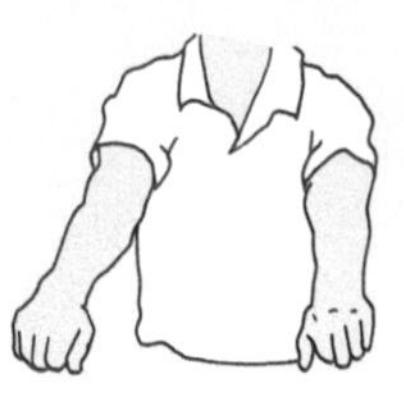

arm abduction -away from median plane / adduction-towards the median plane -shoulder movement

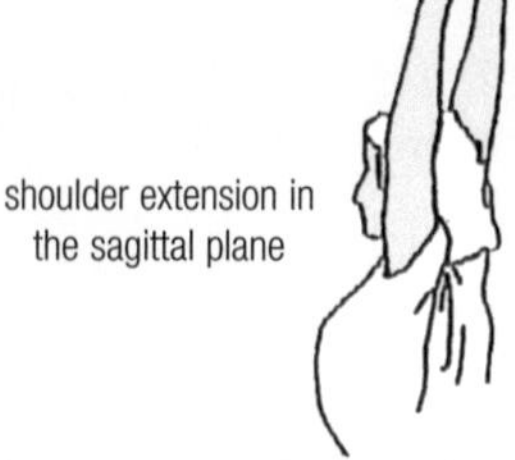

shoulder extension in the sagittal plane

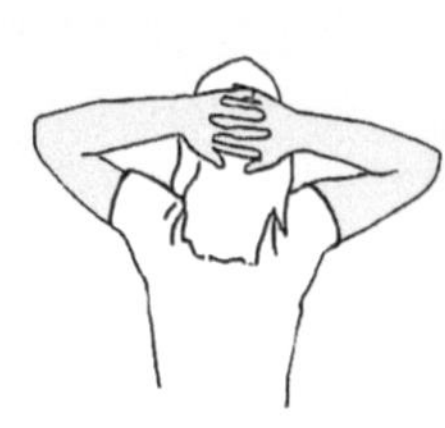

shoulder abduction in the coronal plane (with elbow flexion)

shoulder elevation
- reverse movement shoulder depression
shoulder movement

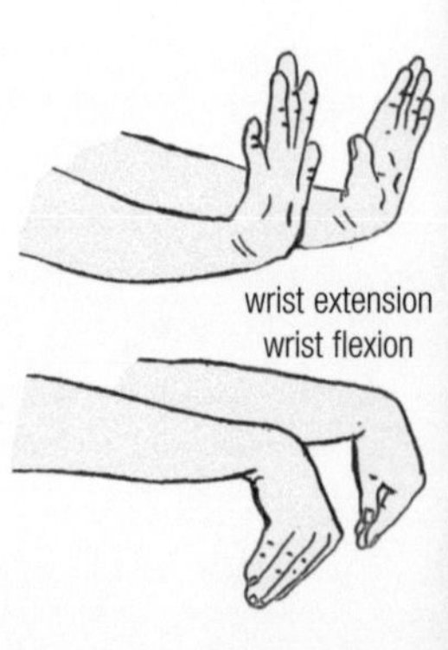

wrist extension
wrist flexion

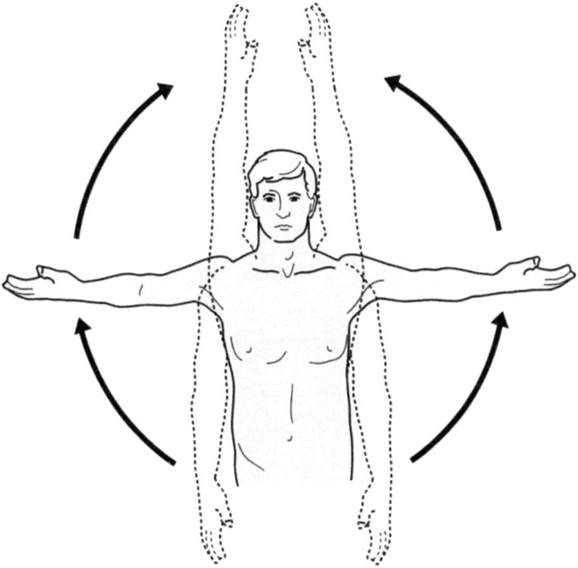

arm/shoulder movements in the coronal plane
commencing from adduction abduction to extension

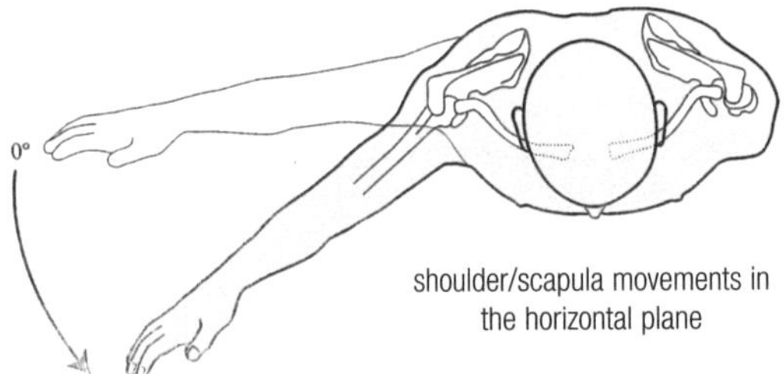

shoulder/scapula movements in the horizontal plane

Map Of Sensory Innervation - Anterior & Posterior

Dermatomes

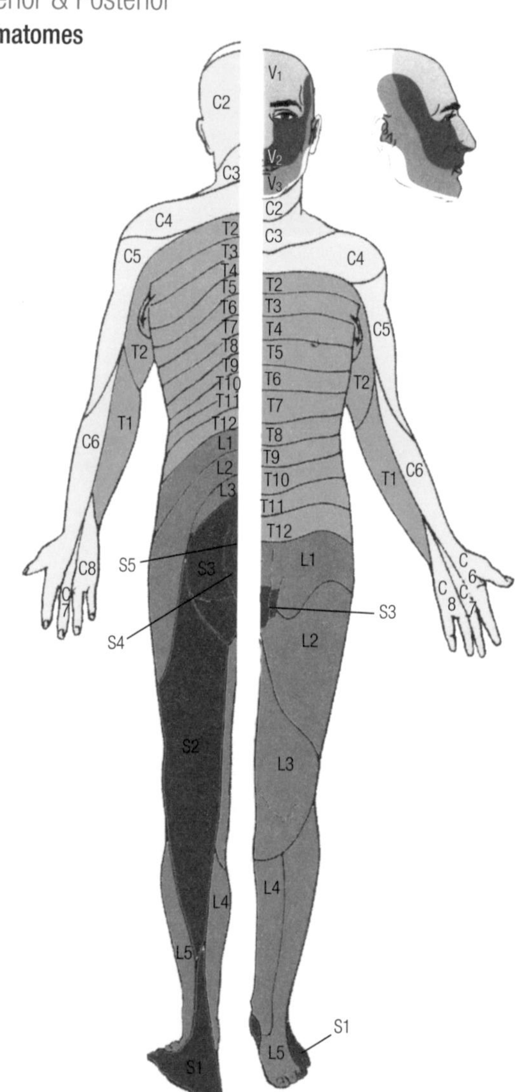

Hand Measurements

Measurements derived from the hand are part of the anthropomorphic measurements (measurements based upon human anatomy). They are helpful to the anatomist as they allow for rough clinical evaluations of surface anatomy w/o having to resort to more complex instruments -

Some other useful measurements have also been included.

9 of these measurements are included in the Vitruvian man.

cubit = 18 ins = 6 palms = elbow to fingertips = forearm + hand
digit < finger = fingertip (1)
ell = 45 ins = 15 palms = arm + body to shoulder
fathom = 72 ins = height
finger = width of finger (2)
foot = length of the shod foot, (longer than the bare foot)
hand = 4 fingers knuckle to knuckle = 4 ins (3)
inch = 25.4 mm = 1/12 part of … a foot
= thumb (i.e. width of at the nail base)
palm = 4 digits =3 inches =7.63cm (4)
shaftment = 2 palms = fist + outstretched thumb (5)
span = 3 palms = ½ cubit = extended hand (6)
yard = 12 palms = 36ins = arm + half body width

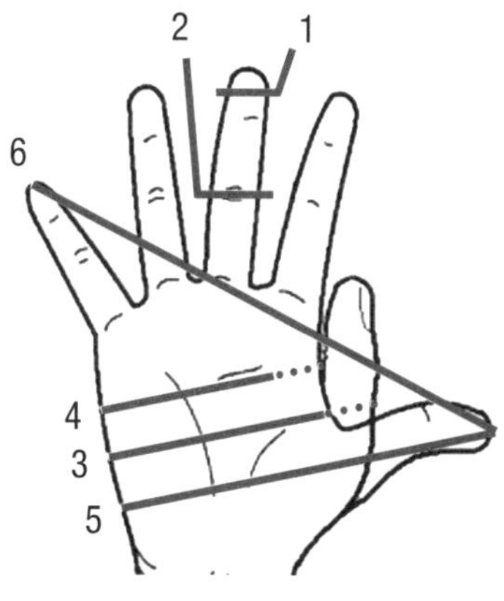

Anatomical Layers

SKIN = EPIDERMIS + DERMIS

EPIDERMIS - consisting of several layers of epithelial cells, which slough off and are replaced b/n 1-7 days - contains all the specialities of the skin: hair, nails sweat glands etc. sitting on supportive layer the basement membrane BM - **burns or wounds to this level may be completely healed without scar formation.**

DERMIS - consisting of connective tissue supplying the epidermis with nerve and blood supply tissue is not replaced except on a needs basis, fairly stable - capable of repair/regeneration contraction (reduction of wound size) and scar formation - **burns or wounds to this level will be detectable and are from tissue replacement not regeneration - scars will not have the properties or the features of the epidermis.**

General properties of the SKIN	THIN / MOBILE
	REGENERATES / REPAIRS
Exceptions PALMS / SOLES	thick skin
SHIN / CHEST	directly over bone
EARS / NOSE	directly over cartilage

SUPERFICIAL FASCIA = LOOSE CONNECTIVE TISSUE + FAT (± Skeletal muscle)

Loose CONNECTIVE TISSUE (CT) + FAT + Skeletal muscle
Not arranged as specific layers - very variable thickness females >males

Gives the intrinsic shape of the body i.e. main deposit of fat determines the FIGURE. Allows for facial expressions.

Networks of Blood Vessels (BV) + Nerves (N) + Lymphatics spread thoughout the area.

This is the point of mobility of the skin.
The point of determining the looseness or tightness of the tissue.
This is the plane used by the plastic surgeons.

Wounds to this area will not alter the function of the tissue underneath. (unless there is excessive contraction).
There may be changed appearance.
There should not in the long term be alteration in sensation.

DEEP FASCIA = CONNECTIVE TISSUE + NEUROVASCULAR TISSUE

Defined anatomical layer - Easily separates from the tissue above. Layers of varying thicknesses and strengths. Acts as a conduit for the Blood and Nerve supply to the deep tissues, particularly the skeletal muscle tightly bound over muscle / anchor for intermuscular septa
CT + BV + N + Lymphatics

MUSCLE & BONE - limbs / appendicular skeleton - VISCERA - Cranium, Thorax, Abdomen and Pelvis / axial skeleton

Organ Weights and Measurements

Organ	Normal Adult Range grams	% of Total Body Weight
Adrenals	12-20 /per gland	-
Brain	1250-1500	2.2
Heart	225-375	0.5
Kidneys	120-200 /per kidney	0.5
Liver	1,500-1,800	2.7
Lungs	250-500 /per lung	1.5
Prostate	20 (>25BPH)	
Spleen	100-250 (may be >800 if exposed to a parasite e.g. malaria)	0.2
Thyroid	15-40 (may be 80 in a "normal" goiter)	-

For more details please see **The A to Z of Organ Anatomy.**

Anatomical Descriptions

How to desribe features in Anatomy Systematically

Joints

classify their type -...	fibrous / cartilaginous / synovial
name the bones involved -...	describe their shapes / and articular coverings
name the ligaments involved -...	capsule / capsular thickenings / accessory / intracapsular
name other intracapsular structures -	synovial membrane / discs / tendons / fat pads / bones
describe functional aspects -...	movements (list muscles involved) stability (list ligaments, bones and relevant muscles) relate the joint to the line of weight
describe their blood supply	
describe their nerve supply	
list the surrounding bursae	
list their relations -...	....superior / inferior / anterior / posterior / laterally / medially

describe any particular radiological feature including CT scan

Organs

define the organ	
describe the general outline -...	shape / size (inc weight) / colour / surfaces (including impressions) / consistency / location (including orientation)
list any functional aspects -...	endocrine / exocrine / autonomic / immunological / physiological / structural / psychological
describe the blood supply	
describe the nerve supply	
describe the lymphatic drainage	
list the relations -...	superior / inferior / anterior / posterior / laterally / medially

describe the Histology and Embryology
describe any particular radiological feature including CT scan

Vessels and Nerves

list in order - origin/course/termination/relations and branches

Muscles

describe their attachments
describe their actions
describe their blood supply
describe their nerve supply
list any unusual features

for more details see
The A to Z of Basic Anatomical Concepts and Anatomical Mapping.

Degrees, Diplomas, Postnominals and other Qualifications, specifically medical.

STYLE GUIDE

1 full stops should not be used in abbreviations of degrees or other qualifications.

2 use either a full or shortened term but not a mixture of both Order of qualifications is:
- i national and royal honours (AO, AM, etc.)
- ii Degrees, Diplomas and then Certificates in conferring order
- iii Fellowships before Memberships
- iv parliamentary designations last.

3 do not place a comma b/n the first postnominal and the person's name, and only use commas b/n different postnominals not b/n several postnominals of the same type i.e. not b/n masters and bachelors degrees.

4 do not place degrees on the same line as the name, only national and royal honours

5 higher degrees absorb lower ones if they are from the same institution.

6 most colleges and institutes do not have recognized abbreviations and so have their name spelt out in full, exceptions CAE = college of advanced education; IT = institute of education; IAE = institute of advanced education.

Abbreviations of common medical qualifications

Abbreviation	Qualification/Membership
B	Bachelor Degree in…
	A 3 year University qualification in various disciplines - increasingly degrees are taking 4 years to complete
BM BS	Bachelor of Medicine Bachelor of Surgery *see MBBS / MBBCh commonly termed "medical degree".
BMedSc	Bachelor of Medical Science
BSc	Bachelor of Science
C	Certificate in …..
	Generally a year qualification.
D	Diploma of …
	Generally a 2 year tertiary qualification. Frequently at a tertiary college. Ma ybe at a postgraduate level.
	Doctorate of ….
	Generally a postgraduate professional degree similar to a PhD but often internally awarded and may not be examined externally. Unlike a PhD standards vary from institute to institute and all Doctorates are not universally recognized as opposed to the PhD.
DDR	Diploma of Diagnostic Radiology
DLO	Diploma of Laryngology and Otorhinology
DM	Doctorate of Medicine
DO	Diploma of Ophthalmology

DPM	Diploma of Psychological Medicine
DS	Doctorate of Science
DTR	Diploma of Radiological Medicine
DPhil	Doctorate of Philosophy of a particular discipline
F	**Faculty of ……** **Generally denoting a group of Departments with a common theme, with faculty members.**
	Fellowship in …. **Generally denoting a "fellowship" in a college as opposed to a "membership".** **Fellows are awarded membership on the basis of qualifications and nominations.**
FACBS	Fellow in the Australian College of Biomedical Scientists
FACD	Fellow of the Australian College of Dermatologists
FACLM	Fellow in the Australian College of Legal Medicine
FACRM	Fellow of the Australian College of Rehabilitation Medicine
FFARCS	Fellow in the Faculty of Anaethetists in the Royal College of Surgeons
FRACO	Fellow in the Royal Australian College of Ophthalmologists
FRACS	Fellow in the Royal Australian College of Surgeons
FRACMA	Fellow in the Royal Australian College of Medical Administration
FRACOG	Fellow in the Royal Australian College of Obstetricians and Gynaecologists
FRACP	Fellow in the Royal Australian College of Physicians
FRACR	Fellow in the Royal Australian College of Radiologists
FRANZCP	Fellow in the Royal Australian and New Zealand College of Psychiatrists
FRC Psych	Fellow in the Royal College of Psychiatrists

Abbreviations of common medical qualifications

FRC Path	Fellow in the Royal College of Pathologists
FRCOG	Fellow in the Royal College of Obstetrics and Gynaecology
FRCPA	Fellow in the Royal College of Pathologists of Australia
FRCR	Fellow in the Royal College of Radiology
FRCS	Fellow in the Royal College of Surgery
Hons	**Honours** **Generally placed after a degree denoting either an additional time of study or an excellent result in the degree. In some universities this may be awarded automatically on completion of a degree.**
M	**Master of …..** **Generally denoting a postgraduate degree of at least 2 years duration, which may or may not be externally examined. In some universities this is awarded as an honorary degree e.g. Oxford.** **Medicine/Medical**
	Member of ….. **Generally denoting membership to a college as opposed to a fellowship**
MB BS	Bachelor of Medicine Bachelor of Surgery* See BM MS / MBBCh
MD	Doctor of Medicine
MS	Master of Surgery
MGO	**Master of Gynaecology and Obstetrics**
MRCP	**Member of the Royal College of Physicians of the Royal Kingdom**
MRCOG	**Member of the Royal College of Obstetrics and Gynaecology**
PhD	**Doctor of Philosophy of a particular discipline**

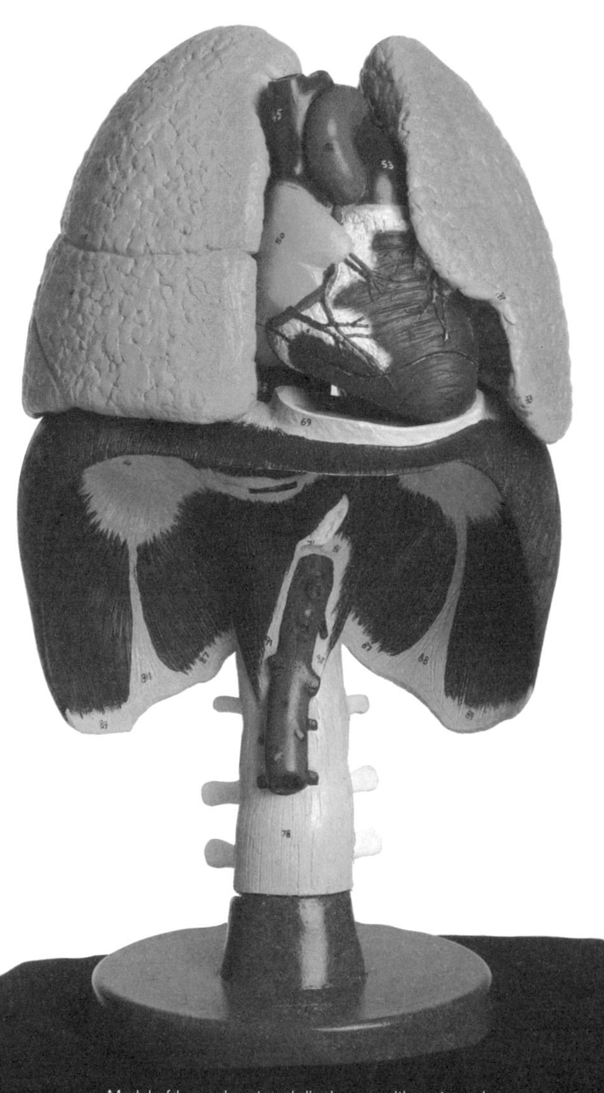

Model of lungs, heart and diaphragm with aorta and oesophagus entering the abdominal cavity.

Common Abbreviations and Terminology guide in academic / university use

AC-	**Australian Centre of …**
	Australian College of …
ACA	Australian Centre for Astrobiology
ACAC	Centre for Advanced Computing – Algorithms & Cryptography
ACANS	Australian Centre for Ancient Numismatic Studies
ACEM	Australasian College for Emergency Medicine
ACEP	Australian College of Emergency Physicians
ACES	Australian Centre for Educational Studies
ACLM	Australasian College of Legal Medicine
ACLS	Advanced Cardiac Life Support course
ACUADS	Australian Council of University Art and Design Schools, the peak body of university visual arts, crafts and design. ACUADS represents over 30 Australian University and TAFE art and design faculties, schools and departments. The Council undertakes leadership, advocacy, policy development, research and community service for the sector, and hosts an active conference and seminar program.
ACU National	**Australian Catholic University National – Brisbane, Canberra, Strathfield, North Sydney, Ballarat and Melbourne**
ADFA	**Australian Defence Forces Academy**
AF	application form
AFTRS	Australian Film Television and Radio School
AHEIA	Australian Higher Education Industrial Association
AIESEC	Association Internationale des Etudiants en Sciences Economiques et Commerciales. The world's largest student organisation. AIESEC is a global network of 50,000 members across more than 83 countries and

	territories at more than 800 universities worldwide. AIESEC facilitates international exchange of thousands of students and recent graduates each year. whether in a paid traineeship or as a volunteer for a non-profit organisation.
Alma Mater	***Nourishing mother.*** The expression is used usually in relation to a person's school, college or university.
Alumni	Alumni - most schools and universities have an office which keeps in contact with graduates and past students and or staff. Useful for creating a network of old students and for fund raising.
AMA	Australian Medical Association
AMDA	Association of Medical Doctors in Asia
AMEE	Association for Medical Education in Europe
AMET	**Australian Mineral Exploration Technologies**
AMIS	**Academic Management Information System**
AMSA	Association of Medical Students in Asia
AMSE	Association of Medical Schools in Europe
APA	**Australian Postgraduate Award**
APS	Academic Program Section
ARC	**Australian Research Council**
ARC Grant	Australian Research Council Grant
ARIES	Australian Research Institute in Education for Sustainability. Australian Research Institute in Education for Sustainability (ARIES) based at Macquarie University. ARIES is the first national institute devoted to the research of education for sustainability and has been established with funding from the Federal Government.
ASCS	Australian Society for Classical Studies
ASEM	Australasian Society for Emergency Medicine
ASM	Australian Society of Microbiology

ATF	**Attach to file**
ATF NFA	**Attach to file no further action**
ATN	The Australian Technology Network (ATN) is a coalition of 5 Australian universities that share a common focus on the practical application of tertiary studies and research. The network claims they have a special strength in the way each of the member universities is focused on producing practical outcomes through their academic activity. The result is graduates and research that is closely aligned to the needs of industry and the wider society. These universities share a common background in the way they distinguished themselves as technical colleges before becoming accredited universities. The member universities of this network are: CIT - Curtin University of Technology, SAIT - South Australian Institute of Technology = University of South Australia, RMIT- Royal Melbourne Institute of Technology University, UTS - University of Technology Sydney, and QIT Queensland Institute of Technology.
AUC	Apple User Consortium
AUQA	Australian Universities' Quality Agency
AVCC	Australian Vice-Chancellors' Committee
BGO	Buildings and Grounds Office
C4ISR	**Command Control Communications Computers Intelligence Surveillance and Reconnaissance (US Pentagon term) covering weapons, strategic planning and force structure.**
CA	Card of Acceptance
CC	Card of Confirmation
CCC	Constitution Credential Committee
CAG	Computer Administrators Group
CAL	**Copyright Agency Ltd**
CAMEC	Cardiac Arrest Medical Emergency course
CBB	**National Key Centre for Biodiversity & Bioresource**

CBR	**Chemical Biological Radiation**
CCS	Critical and Cultural Studies
CDM	Document Management program
CDO	Career Development Office
CDU	**Charles Darwin University (Formerly NTU - Northern Territory University). In 2004, Darwin's Northern Territory University merged with Alice Springs' Central College to form Charles Darwin University - a secondary and tertiary education provider with 9 campuses and centres across the Northern Territory.**
CEO	**Chief Executive Officer = Vice-Chancellor (in a university) see VC**
CFL	Centre for Flexible Learning
Chaplaincy	University life can be very rich and rewarding, as well as challenging and occasionally overwhelming. The aim of the
Chaplains	Chaplaincy Centre is to support students, staff and faculty through all the ups and downs of the university experience.
CIC	Centre for International Communication
CIMS	**Critical Incident Monitoring Study in Emergency Medicine**
CLA	Centre for Lasers and Applications
CLSL	Centre for Language in Social Life
CLT	Centre for Language Technology
CM	**Content Management**
CNMC	Campus Network Management Committee
CoACT	Centre of Australian Category Theory
COE	Centre for Open Education
COE	Council of Europe
COLIS	Collaborative Online Learning and Information Services
Collusion	**Collusion is a form of plagiarism. It may be defined as the unauthorised and unattributed collaboration of**

	students or others in a piece of assessed work.
Council	University Council
CPD	Centre for Professional Development
CPME	Standing Committee of European Doctors
CPSU	Community and Public Sector Union
CQU	**Central Queensland University**
CRC	Marsupial Cooperative Research Centre
CRF	**Central Records File – Central Records was the preceding agency of Records and Archives Services**
CSU	**Charles Sturt University – living success**
CUDOS	Centre for Ultrahigh-Bandwidth Devices for Optical Systems
CUTSD Project	**Teaching and Learning of Greek and Latin in Australian Universities**
Cyber-Plagiarism	**(aka Internet Plagiarism) Use of the Internet to "cut and paste" information to complete assignments.**
Cyber-sloth	**Any student or academic who if they can not find information in cyberspace, do not look for it elsewhere such as in a dictionary, encyclopedia, textbook or a professional journal.**
DCM	**Document & Content Management**
DCMS	Department of Contemporary Music Studies
Deakin	**Deakin University - grow with us, Deakin University aims to be Australia's most progressive University**
Dean	Deans provide academic leadership within a Division/Faculty. Each Division/Faculty is the guardian of programmes (degrees, diplomas and other qualifications) in which students enrol. Generally there is an administrative structure devoted to protecting the office of the Dean.
DEETT	**Disaster External Emergency Team Training**
DEFS	Division of Economic and Financial Studies
Dep Reg	**Deputy Registrar**

DEST	Commonwealth Department of Education, Science and Training (Formerly DETYA - Department of Education, Training and Youth Affairs)
DGB	**Degree Granting Body**
Division	**= Faculty Some universities have Divisions and others Faculties. Interchangeable terms.**
DVC	**Deputy Vice-Chancellor (There are 3 at Macquarie – Academic, Administration, & Research)**
EAP	**English for Academic Purposes**
EB	**Enterprise Bargaining / executive board**
EBL	Evidence based learning
ECOSOC	UN Economic and Social Council
E-Cheating	**The practice of finding and downloading papers from websites. See below - Plagiarism, Paper Mills (aka the cheating game, e-cheating, cut and paste 101)**
ECU	**Edith Cowan University**
EDRM	Electronic Document & Records Management
EDRMS	Electronic Document & Records Management System
EEO	**Equal Employment Opportunity**
EEX	Electronic Exchange
EFT	**Equivalent Full Time**
EFTSU	**Equivalent Full Time Student Unit**
ELS	Emergency Life Support (course)
ELS	Environmental and Life Sciences
EMSA	European Medical Students' Association
EMST	Early management of severe trauma
EPSA	European Pharmacy Students Association

EYF	European Youth Forum
FABLS	**Fluorescence Applications in Biotechnology and Life Sciences**
FAMSA	**Federation of African Med Students' Association**
FATSIL	**Federation of Aboriginal & Torres Strait Islander Languages (Corporation)**
FC	Financial Committee
Federation Fellowship	Federation Fellowships - Australian Research Council awards designed to develop and retain Australian skills The fellowships are regarded as innovative and highly prestigious. They were established under the Australian Government's 2001 innovation action plan, Backing Australia's Ability.
Flagship Grant	Flagship Grants are for teaching development to support a small number of substantial projects contributing to strategies indicated in the Teaching and Learning Plan, which involve significant innovation or developments that will result in improvements to the quality of teaching, student learning or assessment across whole programs or sequences of units. A direct cash contribution from the Division(s)/Departments(s) concerned is a requirement of funding.
FMIS	**Financial Management Information System**
FOI	**Freedom of Information - FOI is the opposite of secrecy. It means the doors and files of government are open and available to the public, instead of being closed to all but a select few. Freedom of information is an important tool for the realisation of democratic goals.**
FOI Act	Freedom of Information Act - The NSW Freedom of Information Act confers on a person a legally enforceable right of access to information held in an agency's records, a right to have official information relating to them amended where it is incomplete, incorrect or misleading and a right to have made known to them the reasons for decisions that have materially affected them.
FOI Officer	Freedom of Information Officer
FORC	Field of Research Concentration

Fulbright Exchange Program	The Fulbright Exchange Program was established in 1946 as an initiative of Senator J. William Fulbright of the USA. Following the end of World War II he was committed to the ideal that mutual understanding through international education and exchange would 'find ways and means of living in peace'. The Fulbright program has promoted educational and cultural exchange between America and over 140 countries throughout the world over the past 50 years. The Australian Fulbright program was established through a Binational Treaty in 1949. Since then almost 2,500 Australians and over 1,700 Americans have been awarded prestigious Fulbright scholarships to study, research and travel in the respective countries. Each year, up to 25 awards are made to Australian Post-Graduates, Post-Doctoral Fellows, Professionals and Senior Scholars. Awardees range from the traditional fields of law, engineering and science to the visual and performing arts. Applications for Australian scholarships open on June 1 and close on August 31 each year.
GA	General Assembly
GDS	Graduate Destination Survey
GEMOC	ARC National Key Centre for Geochemical Evolution and Metallurgy of Continents
GHC	Global Health Council
Go8	**The Group of Eight (Go8) markets itself as the group of 'Australia's Leading Universities'. Membership of the Group of Eight (Go8) includes Adelaide University, The Australian National University, The University of Melbourne, Monash University, The University of New South Wales, The University of Queensland, The University of Sydney, and The University of Western Australia. AKA sandstone universities.**
GPA	**Grade Point Average**
Griffith	**Griffith University – excellence, equity, innovation. Get smarter**
GS	General Secretariat
GSE	Graduate School of the Environment
GSM	Graduate School of Management

Gumtree University	**Term attributed to *The Enterprise University: Power, Governance and Reinvention in Australia* Simon Marginson and Mark Considine - more recently up-springing and fast-growing Australian universities.**
GUSTO	(study)global utilization of Streptokinase and TPA for occluded Coronary arteries.
Head of School	The role of each Head of School is to provide academic and management leadership to the School. This involves strategic planning, managing the people and resources of the School and management of teaching and research programmes, including quality assurance.
Heads of Agreement	**A non-binding document outlining the main issues relevant to a tentative partnership agreement. It is the draft used by lawyers when drawing up the contract. It serves as a guideline for both parties before any documents are ratified.**
HECS	**Higher Education Contribution Scheme**
HRIP Act	**Health Records and Information Privacy Act**
HUSTLE	*First rule of the con: you can't cheat an honest man; you must find someone who wants something for nothing and give them nothing for something.*
IADS	International Association of Dentist Students
ICA	**International Council on Archives**
ICBS	**International Committee of the Blue Shield**
ICROM	**International Centre for the Study of the Preservation and Restoration of Cultural Property**
ICEM	International Conference on Emergency Medicine
ICOM	**International Council on Museums**
ICOMOS	**International Council on Monuments and Sites**
IDP	Education Australia Limited is a global organisation with more than 101 offices in some 55 countries. Owned by 38 prestigious universities in Australia and representing all education sectors, IDP is an independent not-for-profit organisation.

IELTS **International English Language Testing System**

IFLA **International Federation of Library Associations and Institutions**

IFMSA **International Federation of Medical Students' Associations**
The International Federation of Medical Students' Associations (IFMSA) is an independent, non-governmental and non-political federation of medical students' associations throughout the world. In 2004-2005 IFMSA had 92 members, National Member Organizations from 88 countries on six continents and represented more than 1 million medical students worldwide.

IM **Information Management**

IMET International Medical Education

Inforensics **(aka Digital detective work)Instead of dusting for fingerprints, experts in inforensics, short for information forensics, sift through computer files. In today's digital world, you are leaving digital evidence or a digital trail.** *You're actually leaving more of a trail when you go online than you would anywhere else.*

IO **International Office**

IP **Intellectual Property**

IPPNW International Physicians for the Prevention of Nuclear War

IPSF International Pharmacy Student Federation

IRU Australia Innovative Research Universities Australia (IRU Australia) is a group of 6 universities that share a common mode of operation. The group believes that they will be able to establish research concentrations and investment across the universities. The member universities of IRU Australia are: Flinders University, Griffith University, La Trobe University, Macquarie University, Murdoch University and the University of Newcastle.

ISAS **International Society of Aeromedical Services**

ITS International Triage Scale

Ivy League	Ivy League - (a league of universities and colleges in the north-eastern United States that have a reputation for scholastic achievement and social prestige) its 8 members (Brown, Columbia, Cornell, Dartmouth College, Harvard, Penn - University of Pennsylvania, Princeton, and Yale) are highly selective colleges for admission but originally the designation "Ivy League" only refer to their membership in a common athletic conference.
JCU	**James Cook University**
JRCASE	**Joint Research Centre for Advanced Systems Engineering**
LC	Local Committee
LEO	Local Exchange Officer
LMO	local medical officer / locum
LO	Liaison Officer
LOME	Local Officer for Medical Education
LORA	Local Officer of Reproductive Health & AIDS
LORE	Local Officer on Research Exchange
LORP	Local Officer on human Rights and Peace
LPO	Local Public Health Officer
MAMS	Meta access management system. The MAMS project will conduct leading-edge R&D for the integration of multiple solutions to managing authentication, authorisation and identities, together with common services for digital rights, search services and metadata management.
MLS	Medicolegal society
MOU	**Memorandum of Understanding**
MSF	Medecins sans Frontieres
MSI	The Medical Student International
Multi Faith	**The Griffith University Multi-Faith Centre established on the Nathan Campus on the edge of Toohey Forest,**

Centre	overlooks the surrounding suburbs and the mountains beyond. The Multi-Faith Centre provides a venue where people from different religious backgrounds can further their education in their own tradition and participate in multi-faith dialogue. The building provides a number of spaces for prayer, reflection and participation in religious practices. The Centre is also a place where members of Aboriginal and Torres Strait Islander communities can meet, maintain culture and offer education to the wider community on significant issues.
NAS	National Art School
NCELTR	National Centre for English Language Teaching & Research
NGO	Non-Governmental Organisation
NHMRC	National Health and Medical Research Council
NHRC	Risk Frontier - Natural Hazards Research Centre
NMO	National Member Organisation
NOME	National Officer on Medical Education
NORA	National Officer on Reproductive Health & AIDS
NORE	National Officer on Research Exchange
NORP	National Officer on human Rights and Peace
Notre Dame Australia	The University of Notre Dame Australia has campuses in Fremantle and Broome. Notre Dame declares itself to be one of Australia's most exciting and innovative universities. It was founded in 1990 in WA. It is inspired by one of the greatest Catholic universities in the world, the University of Notre Dame in the United States.
NTEU	National Tertiary Education Union
NUS	National Union of Students
OC	Organising Committee
OH & S	Occupational Health and Safety
OLA	Open Learning Agency of Australia

OPTIVA	**Outpatient Intravenous Therapy Association**
Oxbridge	***Noun*** **:(British) general term for an ancient and prestigious and privileged university (especially Oxford or Cambridge Universities) - A short way of referring to Oxford and Cambridge universities.**
Paper Mills	**Websites which sell pre-written dissertations, essays, research papers, and term papers to students (aka Research Paper Mills or Cheat Sites).**
PBL	**Problem Based Learning**
PC	**Project Coordinator**
PCE	**Papyri from the Rise of Christianity in Egypt. A project of the Ancient History Documentary Research Centre [Formerly Corpus Papyrorum Christianarum]**
PELS	**Postgraduate Education Loans Scheme**
PPIPA	**Privacy and Personal Information Protection Act 1998 (NSW)**
Pro Vice-Chancellor	A Pro Vice-Chancellor (PVC) is a senior academic leader of the University who also has senior strategic University-wide management responsibilities. A PVC may oversee a number of Heads of School and/or may oversee a specific Unit or have a University-wide area of responsibility. The PVC manages staff directly reporting to the office of the PVC. PVCs are members of the Senior Management Team (SMT) and report to the Vice-Chancellor.
PVC	Pro Vice-Chancellor
PWG	Permanent Working Group of European Hospital Doctors
RC	Regional Coordinator
QUT	**Queensland University of Technology – a university for the real world**
RACS	Royal Australasian College of Surgeons
Rector	Eccl. law. One who rules or governs–a name given to certain officers of the Roman church. Dict. Canonique, h.v. (Also defined as a guider, leader, director, ruler, and master). At **Tel Aviv University** the Rector is the highest-ranking academic official in the University, subordinate only to the Senate, and he/she serves as the permanent chair for

	Senate meetings. At the **University of Aberdeen** the post of rector dates back to the foundation of the University in 1495, and has been, since 1860, the students' representative on the University Court. Rectors serve for three years and appoint to the Court a Rector's Assessor; the President of the Students' Association further serves student's interests on the Court ex-officio. The Rector plays an important role in representing and supporting the students at the University. The Rector is a position that is independent of both the Students' Association and University administration, allowing the Rector a direct relationship with the students. One of the principal duties is to chair the University Court, at which all major decisions are taken. This ensures that, combined with the President of the Students' Association and the Rector's Assessor (her representative within the University) there is effective student representation at Court. On a day-to-day level, the Rector holds regular surgeries to which any student who would like to raise a particular issue or concern is welcome to come. The Rector also spearheads wider campaigns, both within the University and nationally; to ensure that student life at Aberdeen continues to meet the needs of all students. A Rector and Vice-Chancellor administers the **University of Ottawa**.
Registrar	Registrar and Vice-Principal
RM	Regional Meeting
RM	**Records Management**
RNSH	Royal North Shore Hospital
RPAH	Royal Prince Alfred Hospital
RRTMR	**Research and Research Training Management Plan Reports**
RS	**Re-submit (file) an officer or officer's name will be specified along with the date. This can sometimes be shown as numbered points giving the sequence of who should receive the file.**
Sandstone University	**See Go8**
SANEYOCOP	South Asian Network for Young Conservation Professionals

SC	Standing Committee
SCOME	Standing Committee on Medical Education It is a forum for active discussion for medical students interested in developing medical education. The overall goal is the implementation of an optimal learning environment for all medical students around the world.
SCOPE	Standing Committee on Professional Exchange It is the largest committee within IFMSA. More than 6000 students worldwide participate in the programme each year.
SCOPH	Standing Committee on Public Health Its importance is to make public health issues in medical education and more prominent to the profession and the community. Its aim is to promote an healthy lifestyle through the eradication of smoking, improvement in diet and increasing physical activity.
SCORA	Standing Committee on Reproductive Health including AIDS It aims to raise awareness among medical students about Reproductive Health including sexual education, gender equity, sexual violence, as well as Sexually Transmitted Infections.
SCORE	Standing Committee on Research Exchange. It allows students interested in medical research the possibility to experience research work in a foreign country.
SCORP	Standing Committee on human Rights and Peace. It deals with the problems faced by displaced people and participates in relief efforts. SCORP also works for the prevention of conflicts and human rights abuses.
SCU	**Southern Cross University**
Senate	Academic Senate
SES	Student Enquiry Service
SG	Secretary General
SSEC	Society for the Study of Early Christianity
Swinburne	**Swinburne University of Technology – education that works**

TAF	Travel Assistance Fund
TDC	Technical Data Card
TER	**Tertiary Entrance Rank (replaced by UAI)**
TFN	**Tax File Number**
TOM	Team of Officials Meeting
TRIM	Tower Records and Information Management
Turnitin	Web-based plagiarism detection system - The online system, called Turnitin, compares students' assignments to those of their classmates, previous students from Macquarie and other universities, with material available on the Internet, and with both freely available and subscription-based electronic journals - altogether billions of pages of text. The day after the assignment is submitted, the lecturer is emailed a report highlighting any non-original content in the student's work. The online system will supplement, rather than replace, the University's existing plagiarism policy.
U3A	**University of the Third Age**
UAC	**Universities Admission Centre**
UAI	**University Admissions Index**
U-Can	**University of Canberra**
UN	United Nations
UNAIDS	Joint United Nations Programme on HIV/AIDS
UNDP	United Nations Development Programme
UNE	**University of New England**
UNESCO	**United Nations Educational, Scientific and Cultural Organisation**
UNEVOC	**International Project on Technical and Vocational Education**
UNFPA	United Nations Population Fund
UNHCR	United Nations High Commission for Refugees

UNICEF United Nations Children's Fund
Uni **University**
UniSA **University of South Australia – experience the difference**
UNS **Unified National System - a term used to describe the higher education industry after the abolition of the "binary divide" between universities and colleges of advanced education**
UNSW **University of New South Wales, *UNSW A Portrait* by Professor Patrick O'Farrell, covers the first fifty years of UNSW's history.**
UoW **University of Wollongong – Excellence in Education since 1951**
UQ **University of Queensland**
USC **University of the Sunshine Coast**
USQ **University of Southern Queensland**
USS **Undergraduate Studies Section (in common usage)**
USyd **University of Sydney**
UTas **University of Tasmania – Nationally Distinctive. (sometimes UniTas)**
UTS **University of Technology, Sydney**
UWA **University of Western Australia**
UWS **University of Western Sydney – bringing knowledge to life**
Varsity **Var´si`ty – Noun - 1. a British abbreviation of `university'; usually refers to Oxford University or Cambridge University or 2. a team representing a college or university – first team,**
VC Vice-Chancellor
VCMC Vice-Chancellor's Management Committee
VCP Village Concept Project
VET **Vocational Education and Training**

VPE	Vice-President for External Affairs
VPI	Vice-President for Internal Affairs
VUT	**Victoria University of Technology**
WFME	World Federation on Medical Education
WFPHA	World Federation of Public Health Associations
WHO	World Health Organisation
WHO-AFRO	WHO Regional Office for Africa
WHO-EMRO	WHO Regional Office for the Eastern Mediterranean
WHO-EURO	WHO Regional Office for Europe
WHO-SEARO	WHO Regional Office for the South-East Asia
WHO-WPRO	WHO Regional Office for the Western Pacific
WMA	World Medical Association
YFJ	Youth Forum Jeunesse

For more details see **The A to Z of Medical and Academic Associations, Abbreviations, Terminology and other Jargon**.
See more details on www.aspenonlinelearning.com